LEGAL AND ETHICAL ISSUES IN HUMAN RESEARCH AND TREATMENT

Psychopharmacologic Considerations

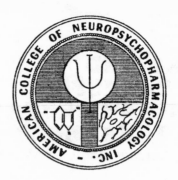

Published under the Imprimatur
of the
American College of Neuropsychopharmacology

LEGAL AND ETHICAL ISSUES IN HUMAN RESEARCH AND TREATMENT
Psychopharmacologic Considerations

Edited by

Donald M. Gallant, M.D.
Professor of Psychiatry
Tulane University School of Medicine
New Orleans, Louisiana

and

Robert Force, LL.M.
Professor of Law
Tulane University School of Law
New Orleans, Louisiana

SP
SP MEDICAL & SCIENTIFIC BOOKS
a division of Spectrum Publications, Inc.
New York • London

Distributed by Halsted Press
A Division of John Wiley & Sons

New York   Toronto   London   Sydney

SPECTRUM PUBLICATIONS, INC.
175-20 Wexford Terrace, Jamaica, N.Y. 11432

Library of Congress Cataloging in Publication Data

Main entry under title:

Legal and ethical issues in human research and treatment—psychopharmacologic considerations.

Papers of a symposium sponsored by the American
College of Neuropsychopharmacology and held in Dec. 17,
1976.
Includes index.
1. Psychopharmacology–Congresses. 2. Psychiatric
ethics–Congresses. 3. Medical research–Law and
legislation--United–Congresses. 4. Informed con-
sent (Medical law)–United States–Congresses.
I. Gallant, Donald M. II. Force, Robert, 1934-
III. American College of Neuropsychopharmacology.
[DNLM: 1. Psychopharmacology--Congresses. 2. Ethics,
Medical--Congresses. 3. Forensic psychiatry--Congress-
es. 4. Human experimentation--Congresses. 5. Research
--Congresses. WM20 L496 1976]
RC483.L38   615'.78'072   72-12628
ISBN 0-89335-039-7

Distributed solely by the Halsted Press Division of John Wiley & Sons, Inc.
New York, New York
ISBN 0-470-26354-7

Contributors

NEIL L. CHAYET, J.D.
Chayet and Sonnenreich
Counsel to the ACNP
Boston, Massachusetts

BURR EICHELMAN, M.D., Ph.D.
Chief of Psychiatry
Veterans Administration Hospital
Director of Laboratory of Behavioral
  Neurochemistry
University of Wisconsin Waisman Center
Madison, Wisconsin

ROBERT FORCE, LL.M.
Professor of Law
Tulane University
School of Law
New Orleans, Louisiana

DONALD M. GALLANT, M.D.
Professor of Psychiatry
Department of Psychiatry
Tulane University
School of Medicine
New Orleans, Louisiana

ANGELA RODDEY HOLDER, LL.M.
Executive Director
Program in Law, Science, and Medicine
Yale University
School of Law
New Haven, Connecticut

ALBERT R. JONSEN, Ph.D.
Associate Professor of Bioethics
Department of Bioethics
Health Policy Program
University of California
School of Medicine
San Francisco, California

KAREN A. LEBACQZ, Ph.D.
Assistant Professor of Christian Ethics
Pacific School of Religion
Berkeley, California

ROBERT J. LEVINE, M.D.
Professor of Medicine and Lecturer in
  Pharmacology
Yale University
School of Medicine
New Haven, Connecticut

RICHARD A. McCORMICK, S.J.
Rose F. Kennedy Professor of Christian
  Ethics
Center for Bioethics
Georgetown University
Washington, D.C.

EDWARD P. SCOTT, J.D.
Staff Attorney
Mental Health Law Project
Washington, D.C.

ALAN A. STONE, M.D.
Professor of Law and Psychiatry
Harvard University
Schools of Law and of Medicine
Cambridge, Massachusetts

We would also like to express our appreciation to Dr. Milton Greenblatt, Dr. Louis Lasagna, Dr. Philip R. May, Dr. Ole J. Rafaelsen, and Dr. Richard J. Wyatt for their contributions in the Commentary sections of this volume.

Contents

Acknowledgments

We wish to express our deep appreciation to all whose efforts and cooperation have made this book possible: to the American College of Neuropsychopharmacology which served as host and sponsoring organization for the symposium on which this book is based: to Linda Terranova for her time and patience in the preparation of the manuscript; and most of all, to Kay Faler, Rochelle Roth, and Leslie Tick for their many hours of editorial assistance which have helped to bring about the prompt publication of this book.

Preface

Science, philosophy, and law appear to be an unlikely trilogy of disciplines to combine in a single presentation at a neuropsychopharmacologic conference. Yet no one who has observed the intrusion of government into the areas of medical treatment and experimentation during the last ten years can fail to perceive the connection. Medical treatment and research, although traditionally subject to a self-imposed conformance to ethical principles, have now become the object of significant legal constraints—including legislation, administrative regulation, and litigation. Standing behind these constraints are the newly awakened and avowed social goals of human dignity and fairness. Briefly stated, the tangible and often valuable fruits of research and treatment must be reconciled with intangible social values, and in some cases yield to them.

This volume, through discussions involving the interplay of science, philosophy, and law, will attempt to construct a projection of what lies ahead for neuropsychopharmacologic research and treatment, not in terms of new drugs, experimental techniques, and treatment modalities, but simply what resolutions are best for our society.

We have divided our inquiry into four major topics, although there is overlap between them. Each topic includes consideration of the past as well as the future. Chapters II and III focus primarily on science and law; Chapters IV and V examine science and ethics. Chapter II involves an analysis of the impact of litigation on psychopharmacologic research and treatment. In Chapter III, legislative and administrative constraints on psychopharmacologic research and treatment are considered. Chapter IV discusses ethical issues in psychopharmacologic research. The final chapter, Chapter V, deals with the ethical issues in psychopharmacologic treatment.

The issues addressed in these papers are not academic. Not long ago, in the spring of 1976, the members of the American College of Neuropsychopharmacology (ACNP), on their own initiative, adopted *A Statement of Principles of Ethical Conduct for Neuropsychopharmacologic Research in Human Subjects,* which is included as the first chapter in this book.[1] In the introduction to the *Statement of Principles* it is stated that: "These Principles are designed to reconcile society's need both for advancing knowledge and for maintaining the dignity and rights of research subjects." Somewhere between the antagonistic extremes of total scientific freedom of action and overly restrictive regulation of research, ethical precepts and legal mechanisms must reconcile and balance the competing interests of society. It is in effecting this reconciliation that many problems are found.

We can consider the two other competing principles: the concepts of equality and freedom of choice. These principles relate to the concept of risks and their distribution. In some experiments with human subjects there are risks, just as there are risks in treatment. How should these risks be distributed in society? It may be suggested that in a just society the risks would be distributed equally. Through a process of randomization, every person in society, for the greater good of society, would assume a duty to be a subject in scientific experiments or to be exposed to new treatment modalities. In contrast, it may also be suggested that in a just society each person should have the choice to expose himself to risk or not. Implicit in this more individualistic approach is a recognition that some people are more intelligent, attractive, healthier, wealthier, etc., than others, and there is no social obligation to attempt to equalize these differences among people. With regard to treatment and experimental risks, the individualistic approach makes no attempt to control individual participation. Therefore, the poor, the institutionalized, the incarcerated, and the students appear disproportionately in experimental subject groups.

While the notion of equality is attractive, so is the concept of freedom of choice. We have not, however, tried to reconcile these competing interests. Instead, a compromise has been arranged. We follow the individualistic-choice approach in the United States, but rather than introduce limited notions of equality or randomization, we have created legal rules that inhibit experimentation or treatment under certain conditions. What we have done, in a

---

[1] Although the *Statement of Principles* has been officially approved by the entire membership of the American Colleges of Neuropsychopharmacology, it should be stated that the following chapters and commentary sections are not intended to represent any additional official positions of the ACNP.

sense, is to draw a line between ethical manipulation of some persons and manipulation that might be characterized as "unjust" use or exploitation. All manipulation may be considered unfair to some degree, but all unfairness need not, in a legal or ethical sense, be considered unjust. The line between ethical and unjust manipulation of humans for research is drawn according to what society is willing to tolerate at the particular time in question. This is not to suggest that there is no bottom line. Despite the fact that in the Nazi society certain inhuman and outrageous experiments on people were tolerated, these were still unjust exploitations. In the United States, our Constitution and its Amendments are intended to protect the individual from possible abuses of the majority.

The difficulties of distinguishing between permissible and unjust use of humans are much more subtle in this country. The pivotal distinction is based on the notion of *consent*. We will not allow exposure of an individual to any experiment without his consent (or that of one legally authorized to give it). Implicit in the doctrine of consent is the notion that the patient or subject must have some understanding of what he is consenting to; hence, consent must be informed. The consent requirement is properly used to maintain a certain level of human dignity which society insists upon. It is a device to prevent a gross overreaching or an unconscionable advantage. In short: the consent doctrine is one device that we use to distinguish between permissible and unjust manipulation in human research and treatment. It is not a device designed to eliminate differences among people—differences that make it easier to recruit "volunteers" from certain classes of people. If we set the requirements of consent below minimal ethical standards, consent becomes a sham and is of no aid in preventing unconscionable exploitation. On the other hand, if the requirements for obtaining informed consent are set too high, we are, in reality, repudiating experiment or treatment. Setting consent requirements that are unrealistic or impossible to comply with, or that destroy the methodological validity of the proposed experiment or treatment, represents a rejection of the individualistic-choice approach. The consent issue should not be the battleground between those who opt for individual choice and those who advocate equality. So long as we adhere to the individualistic-choice approach, consent should be viewed as what it is: a legal tool to prevent unjust and unconscionable exploitation of individuals or groups as medical subjects under certain circumstances. The consent device represents a restriction of the individualistic approach, not a reconciliation of competing views.

A second and related problem involves the use of the legal term "rights." It is fashionable in some circles to discuss scientific problems in terms of patients' rights. Much of the current legal ferment is concerned with the protection of the individual patient's or subject's rights—e.g., the right not to be subject to experimental practices or treatment without having given "fully informed consent," the right to treatment, the right to refuse treatment, etc.

The law does fashion some protection against unjust exploitation that may result in injury, unnecessary pain, or loss of freedom. The vehicle for extending such protection is the creation or recognition of "rights" for subjects and patients. However, we should not approach the subject of rights mechanically or simplistically. The essence of "rights" for the protection of patients and subjects involves a recognition that people should not be singled out arbitrarily and subjected unjustly to measures that are inconsistent with human dignity. It is in this context that a person or group of people, under certain circumstances, may have a right to treatment or a right to refuse treatment, or a right to make an informed choice. This right relates to preserving the subject's or patient's health and dignity.

In some instances, it has been argued that institutions providing residential treatment should be prohibited from compelling patients to work without compensation. Presumably, this position intends to protect the patients' right to compensation, their right against involuntary servitude. Suppose, though, the practical effect of securing this right is the termination of a work therapy program that has proved highly efficacious (as well as low on risk and high on human dignity). It is no answer to say that we should have a work therapy program that includes compensation since the state may not have finances to support this program. If the program is terminated, the patient cannot participate. If the patient cannot participate, has he been denied his right to efficacious treatment? Which right, compensation or efficacious treatment, comports most with the patient's health needs and a recognition of his dignity? What is best for the patient? What would each of us opt for if we were in the position of the patient?

Another example concerns the use of prison inmates as volunteer subjects in research. It has been suggested that inmates should not be permitted to participate as subjects in medical research. This position assumes that all inmate participation is predicated on coercion and that a person has a right not to be coerced into participating in experimental programs. On the other hand, doesn't an inmate have a right to participate in a program that may relate to some illness, disease, or condition that may or may not have been a factor in bringing about his incarceration? Doesn't an inmate have the right to earn money or early release from prison for participating in a research program? Doesn't taking away his opportunity to participate impose additional restrictions on his already restricted life? Again, which approach truly protects the right of the inmate? What is in his best interests? What course would we choose for ourselves?

When the question of "rights" in medical treatment and research is considered from the perspective of the patient or subject, a complex balancing of factors is involved. But these difficult decisions cannot be resolved by examining only the interests of the individual. Both in defining and applying a notion of "rights," there are societal interests that must also be included as a consideration in the balancing process. Individual rights are not absolute. Even in the case of rights expressly protected under the United States Constitution, the common good is customarily taken into account by the Supreme Court in defining the scope of the right and especially in resolving specific conflicts. This concept has been demonstrated in cases involving speech, property, quarantine, etc.

Basic ethical conflicts can also exist between the two important goals of individualized medical treatment and well-designed research with humans. The following are examples of such conflicts. In medical practice it may be unethical to apply a treatment modality whose efficacy has not been shown to be statistically more beneficial than an inert technique; however, the use of randomization in conducting a scientific study for patients in human research to obtain valid, efficacious data is frequently questionable from an ethical viewpoint. It is understood that a research study with humans without using scientific methodology is unethical because it exposes the patient to risks for no valid reasons. However, since the use of additional medications, such as hypnotics for sleep, is contraindicated in certain types of well-controlled psychopharmacologic studies, such a design sacrifices the comfort of the patient to the goal of the research project. Similarly, the use of randomization and double-blind techniques without fully informed consent interferes with the personal relationship between the physician and the patient and thus sacrifices the patient's individual expectations of personal care from his physician.

A conflict also exists between obtaining fully informed consent in an ethical manner and conducting competent research. In most scientific studies with humans, the disclosure of full information would automatically affect the validity of the research results. Complete information, fully explained to the patient prior to a drug study, about the use of randomization, the need to avoid the use of any additional pharmacologic agents during the study, the need to adhere to the protocol design, and the possible use of placebo may not only influence and possibly invalidate the results of the study, but may also seriously hamper the conduct of the study by the refusal of a considerable number of patients to participate in such a project. After receiving such information, many patients' choice of alternative therapies from their own physicians would cause a biased selection of patients for a study whose data could not then be extrapolated to other populations. Only a few studies, such as those projects that evaluate two or more types of therapeutic modalities that may have similar benefits and risks and do not require placebo control, will attract a significant number of patient participants. Thus, it is our opinion that if the present trend toward full disclosure and demonstration of understanding is required without exceptions, competent scientific research in human patients will not be properly performed. If the present trend continues, societal and cultural values will have to change before medical experimentation with humans results in any further significant advances, except for occasional discoveries by either serendipity or genius.

It is said in rebuttal that the present-day trend could be halted if the scientific investigator would assume full responsibility for the clinical trial with "approval of his informed peers" and thereby avoid the necessity of obtaining informed consent since "the subject's only real protection, the public as well as the medical profession must recognize, depends on the conscience and compassion of the investigator and his peers" (1). We strongly object to this statement. There are multiple cases in the literature which reveal that total reliance on the investigator will inevitably lead to some grossly incompetent errors in ethics; it is apparent that the very existence of review committees partically composed of individuals of disciplines outside the scientific organizations should serve to make the investigator more cautious in his approach to research in humans. Basic to the assumption of the need for full information prior to obtaining informed consent is the fact that the physician-investigator regards the research patient as an individual deserving full respect, not to be manipulated without knowledge of the ramifications of his participation. Excepting certain scientific requirements of methodology, any manipulation of the patient without his full knowledge of the methodological procedure is ethically questionable.

Informed consent is the basic prerequisite for all medical treatment and research, and the question of what constitutes informed consent provides the conflicts both in research and treatment. Without informed consent, psychopharmacologic intervention cannot be ethically or legally justified. In those patients considered to be incapable of giving informed consent, the consent must then be obtained from the legally authorized representative as defined by the law of the state in which the patient resides. However, in many cases of informed consent, the procedure becomes a fraud, without either the physician or the lawyer realizing it (2). In one study of consent forms, it was concluded that comprehension and consent to volunteer were inversely related to the length of the form (3). Thus, at times, the greater the attempt of the conscientious investigator to fully inform his patient, the more confused and more mistrustful the patient may become.

It should be stressed that in most areas of psychiatric research, there are no adequate animal models for mental or emotional illness. Therefore, continued experimentation in man is essential if we are to learn the etiology of and formulate the proper treatment for these illnesses. The normal volunteer cannot be used as a model for this type of experimentation; it is apparent that the patient with the specific illness (e.g., the schizophrenic patient with limited mental capacity who is the center of the controversy of informed consent and for whom multiple legalistic approaches have been proposed for proper informed consent) must be the focus of the research.

As methodology in medical research has been improved by research designs emphasizing controls and statistically valid results, the tendency to depersonalize the investigator-patient relationship increases. The introduction of innovative word changes may also contribute to the distortion of traditional values. Substitution of the word "subject" for "human research patient," the use of terms such as "benefit-risk ratio," "institutional review boards" rather than "human research evaluation committees," etc., may tend to minimize the dignity and value of the human being involved in the experiment.

These ethical and legal questions have always been present, but only in the last fifteen years have they been debated in open forums at scientific and legal sessions as well as in the medical-legal literature, magazines, and newspapers. In 1962, there were no statutes in the United States that required proof of efficacy of drugs or offered adequate guidelines for the investigation of these drugs in humans. Investigation of the profits of the pharmaceutical industry and the appearance of the teratogenic effects of thalidomide resulted in the Kefauver-Harris Amendment to the U.S. Pure Food and Drug Law, the first significant amendment to this law since 1938. A major emphasis of this amendment was requirement of proof of efficacy as well as safety of drugs. More adequate data of toxicity in animals and submission of an Investigation of a New Drug (IND) application were required before the drug could be tested in man. More adequate protocols for testing the efficacy of the drug in man were outlined, and more careful evaluation of data was required before a New Drug Application (NDA) could be approved. By 1966, the Federal Drug Administration (FDA) requested the National Academy of Sciences to act as an advisory body to ascertain the efficacy of drugs introduced into therapy between 1938 and 1962. Approximately 4,000 drugs were evaluated, and most of the drug-efficacy decisions were made by 1970. In this case, the use of academic experts by the National Academy of Sciences set a helpful precedent These attempts to correct the negligence of the past finally culminated in the 1974 legislation establishing the National Commission for the Protection of Human Subjects of Biomedical and Behavioral Research (NCPHSBBR). The combination of rapid advances in medical technology, the rise of consumers' movements able to attract national attention, and the increase of lucrative malpractice litigation are among the major factors for the recent stimulation of public interest in the conduct of research and treatment by medical researchers.

The present trend toward increased legal regulation of research and treatment is almost certain to continue indefinitely. Informal standards of professional ethics are no longer respected by the politicians, and even laymen are becoming wary of self-regulation by any organization. Undoubtedly a greater sensitivity to the dignity and rights of research subjects and patients now exists in the United States. However, in most cases, the medical and research establishments have assumed a defensive stand on the problems involving the right to treatment, civil rights of patients, and regulation of the conduct of research.

Recent advances in clinical pharmacology, particularly those rapid advances in clinical psychopharmacology during the 1950s and 1960s, contributed to the development of unrealistic expectations of scientific achievement and an uncritical attitude by the general public. With recent emphasis on patient rights and redistribution of federal priorities from research to services, the public and Congress have now developed cynical, overly critical attitudes toward research and even a distrust of the consequences of scientific advancement. The recent controversy at the Harvard Medical School about the XYY study, the temporary cessation of research with genetic materials at the same institution, and general public misconceptions about the results and goals of treatment with psychoactive agents represent examples of these rapidly changing public and legislative opinions.

The purported conflict between science and the public has been further enhanced, perhaps inadvertently, by some civil libertarians. The promotion of such terms as "patient advocate" instead of "patient surrogate," as inferred by Neil Chayet in Chapter III, only serves to create an "emotional adversary" role for the patient's representative rather than to provide a substitute or deputy for the patient.

Requirements for adequately controlled studies are necessary if we are to devise more efficacious treatment methods for those many millions of individuals suffering from such illnesses as schizophrenia and depression. Public reaction to occasional episodes of gross misconduct and negligence by a few researchers should not be allowed to result in legislative acts and regulatory restraints that unnecessarily hinder the competent researcher from accomplishing his goal. It is hoped that we all share one basic ethical premise: we must abandon the pursuit of knowledge in any area if the human cost of achieving it is too high. However, overly restrictive regulations may discourage researchers from entering the field or remaining in it.

Decisions in medicine, both in research and practice, are made prospectively, while decisions in the courtroom are rendered retrospectively. The obvious difference in foresight and hindsight places the physician-researcher at a disadvantage in the courtroom, but no more so than his patient at the start of the doctor-patient relationship.

The present medical care system in this country, consisting of different modalities of private care, state and city charity care, and several federal systems, provides an inequitable distribution in quality of medical care as well as exposure to research risks. When a medical student performs a spinal tap for the first time on a patient who requires such a procedure—often a traumatic experience for the student as well as for the patient—it is rarely performed on a private patient in a private hospital room. Similar examples often occur without the medical student, teacher, or practitioner of medicine questioning the system; these inequities will continue to exist as long as there is more than one economic system of medical care. Even then, who among us would be willing to join a lottery that would put us at risk to be selected for spinal taps by medical students or to participate as research subjects? Many persons in our society are preoccupied with their individual rights and privileges, but fail to understand that, unless they actively share the responsibility and required risks to promote the welfare of the society, that society will stagnate and eventually disintegrate. It appears that our society would have to undergo a radical transformation of our present values regarding individual rights and *obligations to the society that serves us* before equal access to competent medical care and exposure to research risks would be possible. This transformation may be impossible as well as impractical to accomplish.

Therefore, it is the hope of the editors of this volume that the ethical and legal directions for psychopharmacologic research and treatment presented here will offer practical guidelines for maintaining the primary ethical values of the physician-scientist: obligations to the patient, duty to humanity, and adherence to truth. Our goal should be the maintenance of these primary ethical values for conduct between human beings without seriously hampering the acquisition of scientific knowledge that may prove to be beneficial to both the individual and the society.

D.M. Gallant
R. Force

REFERENCES

1. Ingelfinger, F.J. Informed (but uneducated) consent. *New Eng. J. Med.,* 287:466-470, 1972.
2. Laforet, E.G. The fiction of informed consent. *JAMA,* 235:1579-1585, 1976.
3. Epstein, L.C., and Lasagna, L. Obtaining informed consent: Form or substance. *Arch. Intern. Med.,* 123:682-688, 1969.

LEGAL AND ETHICAL ISSUES IN HUMAN RESEARCH AND TREATMENT

Psychopharmacologic Considerations

CHAPTER I

A Statement of Principles of Ethical Conduct for Neuropsychopharmacologic Research in Human Subjects

It was the opinion of the editors, D.M. Gallant and R. Force, that the adoption of this Statement of Principles by the American College of Neuropsychopharmacology (ACNP) was of sufficient importance to warrant the publication of this ethical code of conduct for research in human subjects as the first chapter in this book, particularly since the contents of this Statement directly relate to the important ethical and legal issues discussed in the subsequent chapters and commentary sections.

The request to develop the Statement of Principles was made by Dr. Philip R. May, President of the ACNP, to Dr. Donald M. Gallant, Chairman of the Ethics Committee, in December 1974. The first and second drafts of this Statement were mailed to twenty-seven people, including all members of the ACNP Council, all members of the Ethics Committee, and other individuals inside and outside of the ACNP who, we believed, would offer additional helpful suggestions because of their diverse professional experiences. We received responses from twenty-four of the twenty-seven individuals, and the majority of the suggestions were incorporated into a third draft. The third draft was mailed to the entire voting membership in September 1975, and the open meeting on this draft was conducted Thursday, December 18, 1975, at the annual meeting of the ACNP. The fourth and fifth (final) drafts were formulated from the suggestions and advice offered at this meeting and at the subsequent Council meeting on January 9, 1976. The final draft of the

Statement was approved by the membership of the ACNP in a mail ballot in June 1976. Throughout the process of developing the initial draft into a final document, the Chairman of the Ethics Committee received invaluable help and advice from Robert Force, LL.M., and Neil Chayet, J.D.

It was recognized that there was a need for a Statement of Principles that exists independently of standards currently contained in law since governmental regulations may vary over time and some universal standards are necessary for the conduct of all neuropsychopharmacologic research in human subjects. As emphasized in the introduction to the Statement of Principles, the intent of this Statement is that all human research, federally funded or not, and regardless of the source of funds, should be subject to the same principles of ethical conduct.

D.M. Gallant

INTRODUCTION

This *Statement of Principles* is intended to serve as an ethical guide to apply specifically to neuropsychopharmacologic research with human subjects performed by the members of the ACNP. Neuropsychopharmacologic research is here defined as the evaluation of the effects of synthetic compounds or natural products employed as investigational agents that affect the brain and behavior. While the Principles formulated herein may be relevant to other areas of research with human subjects, this *Statement of Principles* was not designed with that broad goal in mind. This *Statement of Principles* is neither to be used as a legal statement nor as a binding legal document, either in a court of law or within the ACNP. It is not intended to be the ultimate statement of ethical principles, but rather a framework for evolving ethical concepts. It should not be used retrospectively to judge research conducted prior to its adoption by the ACNP membership.

To distinguish and clarify various ethical obligations which may be applicable in some research studies and not in others, this *Statement of Principles* employs the following terms to describe various types of subjects:

1. *Patient*—a person who has entered into a doctor-patient relationship with the scientific investigator or another physician in the facility and who is a subject in a research study primarily intended to bring about beneficial changes in the condition for which he is being treated.

2. *Patient-Volunteer*—a patient who is a subject in a research study not primarily intended to bring about beneficial changes in the condition for

which he is being treated, but which may add to the knowledge about emotional and mental disorders.

3. *Nonpatient-Volunteer*—a person who is a subject in a research study primarily intended to benefit society, not the subject himself; however, in certain studies, this person may also benefit.

4. *Subject*—an encompassing term which refers to all persons described in the three previous categories.

Neuropsychopharmacologic research in the past twenty-five years has made significant contributions to human welfare. For example, as a result of the discovery and development of new drugs, patients with severe psychiatric and neurological illnesses, who were once considered untreatable and relegated to overcrowded institutions, have been able to return to their families and communities, often as productive persons. Others have been able to avoid institutionalization or to reduce its duration substantially as a result of drug therapy administered in outpatient treatment programs. However, the imperfections of existing treatment methods require increased scientific efforts to decrease the pain and suffering of patients and their families.

Scientific research does not exist in a vacuum. It should be emphasized that all persons living in society have a moral responsibility to participate in efforts to promote and contribute to the present and future welfare of that society. Research is one of these obligations. Notwithstanding the substantial benefits to society derived from neuropsychopharmacologic research, another societal interest must be considered—the welfare of each research subject. These Principles are designed to reconcile society's need both for advancing knowledge and for maintaining the dignity and rights of research subjects. It should also be recognized that advancement in medical research with subsequent benefit to society is impossible without some risks.

This *Statement of Principles* exists independently of standards currently contained in law or proposed governmental regulations. This independence has significant implications: (1) While law and ethics interrelate, they are by no means identical in that ethical requirements may affect behavior not within legal control. (2) This *Statement of Principles* applies to all neuropsychopharmacologic research in human subjects whether or not the research is presently covered by applicable governmental regulations. (3) Standards of governmental regulations may vary, and there is no assurance that present standards will prevail in the future. (4) Present laws and regulations at times impose bureaucratic controls which restrict research without providing a corresponding increase in protection for the research subject. (5) Professional organizations whose members are concerned with research have had little opportunity to contribute to shaping legal and ethical standards or to provide a model for future regulations of research involving human subjects. (6) Finally, the existence of a *Statement of Principles* provides a reference point for the conduct of neuropsychopharmacologic research in human subjects.

One of the moral obligations of biomedical scientists is the acquisition of knowledge to preserve and enrich life. In accordance with scientific tradition, there are certain identifiable ethical values that should be supported for the maintenance and improvement of society. However, these underlying values are not described specifically in the *Statement of Principles;* instead, it addresses itself to what the scientific investigator must or may do. Implicit in the Principles is the recognition and acceptance of these cardinal ethical values, as exemplified by voluntary consent, consideration of risks versus benefits, avoidance of unnecessary pain or disabling long-term effects, and benefits to both the individual and society.

The Principles are phrased in general terms without enumerating every possible ethical problem. A *Statement of Principles* of such specificity would require volumes, yet would inevitably be incomplete. The general principles expressed in this *Statement* should provide clear standards for resolving specific ethical questions which may arise in the course of neuropsychopharmacologic research and the use of data resulting from such studies.

Important distinctions are made in this *Statement* among various types of human subjects. Notwithstanding the premise that in all research unnecessary harm to the subject should be avoided and that any possible disadvantages which may result should be disclosed to him, the ethical propriety of neuropsychopharmacologic research in any given case also depends on the subject's status as a patient, a patient-volunteer, or a nonpatient-volunteer.

The scientific investigator has certain ethical obligations to a "patient" which are inherently different from those of the researcher to the "patient-volunteer" or the "nonpatient-volunteer" (as these terms are defined above). In studies with patients, the individual patient should reasonably be expected to benefit from the research results. Research studies with volunteers, both patients and nonpatients, should reasonably be expected to produce benefits for society.

Procedures for securing subject consent to participate may depend on whether the subject is incompetent or competent, a child or an adult, or a member of a group particularly vulnerable to undue influence. The resolution of many ethical problems may well depend on the awareness and intelligent application of these distinctions.

The *Statement of Principles,* generally, is phrased in terms of what the scientific investigator must or may do in order to assure ethical requirements. In addition, this *Statement* addresses itself to the qualifications of the scientific investigator and takes the position that any clinical research undertaken by an unqualified investigator is, of itself, unethical behavior.

The *Statement of Principles* adopts the legal distinction between the words "shall" and "may." The word "shall" is used to denote something which is mandatory.

PRINCIPLE 1: *QUALIFICATIONS OF THE SCIENTIFIC INVESTIGATOR*

A scientific investigator, before he assumes full responsibility for conducting neuropsychopharmacologic research studies with human subjects, shall have had adequate training and experience to conduct the research study he proposes.

Commentary

The scientific investigator's prior experience as an assistant in neuropsychopharmacologic studies with human subjects shall be given weight in assessing his competence. The adequacy of the investigator's experience should be a concern of the Institutional Review Board or its equivalent.

PRINCIPLE 2: *DESIGN AND METHODOLOGY OF RESEARCH STUDIES*

A neuropsychopharmacologic research study with human subjects shall be designed and carried out in accordance with generally accepted scientific principles.

Commentary

Experimentation with human subjects without reasonable anticipation of patient benefit or without reasonable anticipation of adding to the body of scientific knowledge is ethically unacceptable. Therefore, no risks can be justified when the experimental design is poor. The scientific investigator has the general obligation to extract the greatest amount of useful information from the smallest number of subjects with minimal risk or discomfort.

The following examples are some of the considerations that should be taken into account in the preparation of research protocols: (1) Subjects should be selected only if they appear suitable to test the specific hypotheses proposed in the research. (2) Whenever feasible, studies should be planned so that the number of subjects in the study is consistent with the statistical requirements necessary to assure that the data obtained or the conclusions drawn are likely to be valid. (3) When appropriate, provision should be made for control or comparison groups, or for subjects who serve as their own controls, to assure that information gathered has potential utility. (4) The investigator should have access to appropriate statistical expertise to assure that the results of his experiment will be meaningful to the scientific community. (5) In research designs of studies in patients, randomization of assignment to treatment should be employed only when the scientific question requires such a procedure and when increased risk to the subject is considered to be minimal.

It is recommended that a letter including a clear statement that approval for the protocol was obtained accompany research papers submitted for publication.

PRINCIPLE 3: *REVIEW AND APPROVAL OF HUMAN RESEARCH STUDIES*

A scientific investigator shall not undertake a neuropsychopharmacologic research study involving human subjects without the approval of an appropriate, qualified reviewing body. The investigator shall ascertain that the reviewing body has specific guidelines for the submission, initial approval, and periodic review of all protocols for research studies with human subjects. Once having secured initial approval, the investigator should obtain subsequent approval for any substantial deviation from the protocol.

Commentary

The organization of Institutional Review Boards for approval and review of research studies with human subjects has been advocated by scientific investigators and required by the United States Department of Health, Education and Welfare (DHEW), as described in the Federal Register, May 30, 1974 (1, 2). In accordance with these guidelines, this committee of the institution sponsoring investigation with human subjects serves to protect the rights and welfare of the participants.

No individual investigator, regardless of his qualifications and competency, is infallible. Thus, both the scientific investigator and the subject benefit from the establishment of review committees, the very existence of which stimulates thoughtfulness and encourages responsibility on the part of the scientific investigator.

A scientific investigator who is not affiliated with an institution which has an Institutional Review Board shall not undertake a neuropsychopharmacologic research study unless it is initially approved and periodically reviewed by an independent review body that is substantially the equivalent of an Institutional Review Board.

In the event that DHEW should ultimately abandon or substantially restrict its requirements for Institutional Review Boards, review and approval of research studies by appropriate review bodies would continue to be required by this *Statement of Prinicples.* Present governmental regulations provide possible exceptions to review of research if it is not federally funded. The intent of this Principle is that all human research, regardless of the source of funds, should be subject to review.

The scientific investigator has the responsibility to serve on an Institutional Review Board or its equivalent, when requested, in order to maintain the necessary principle of review of research by one's peers. If the scientific investigator is a member of an Institutional Review Board which is considering his project, he should not participate in the vote relative to that research project.

Reviewing bodies have an obligation to establish a fair procedure for approval and independent review of their decisions.

PRINCIPLE 4: *RESPONSIBILITIES OF THE SCIENTIFIC INVESTIGATOR AND THE APPLICATION OF THIS STATEMENT OF PRINCIPLES*

Individual Responsibility

Each scientific investigator shall ascertain and consider the current ethical standards applicable to neuropsychopharmacologic research studies with human subjects.

Application of this *Statement of Principles*

1. The scientific investigator shall conduct studies in neuropsychopharmacologic research with human subjects in substantial accordance with the ethical principles contained in this *Statement of Principles*—with respect for subjects and with concern for their dignity, welfare, and rights. This responsibility, in addition, is imposed on all associates, employees, or students who assist the scientific investigator.

2. The scientific investigator shall take reasonable precaution to assure that the Principles contained in this *Statement* are observed by all persons who assist him in the research study.

3. The ethical responsibilities imposed by this *Statement of Principles* shall become applicable when the scientific investigator makes the initial decision to undertake a neuropsychopharmacologic research study with human subjects and shall continue through the conclusion of the research study, including all necessary steps to protect any privileged or confidential material pertaining to subjects in the study.

4. The scientific investigator shall take reasonable precautions to acquaint himself with and adhere to applicable laws and regulations which are relevant to the research study he proposes to undertake. State laws on privileged and confidential material vary; the investigator should acquaint himself with the laws of the state where he resides.

PRINCIPLE 5: *CONSIDERATIONS IN DETERMINING WHO MAY BE A PROPER SUBJECT IN A RESEARCH STUDY; GOAL OF RESEARCH STUDY DETERMINES TYPE OF SUBJECT*

General Responsibilities

The scientific investigator engaged in neuropsychopharmacologic research with human subjects shall take all reasonable precautions for preserving the dignity, rights, and safety of his subjects.

Studies with Patients

1. In neuropsychopharmacologic research involving patients, an anticipated therapeutic effect should be the primary but not necessarily the exclusive goal. The scientific investigator should evaluate the research regimen with a view toward doing no harm to the patient by withholding treatment which has a very high degree of probability of significantly improving the patient's condition. Some research might be designed primarily to make an accurate diagnosis prior to definitive treatment or to develop prognostic indicators for selection of optimal treatment of the patient's disease.

2. Patients who are mentally incompetent should not be subjects in neuropsychopharmacologic research studies which have no diagnostic, therapeutic, or prophylactic goals for the subject except in those cases where there are no "realistic risks" involving long-term side effects or toxicity. Some examples of relatively minor and safe procedures are comparisons of physical measurements, psychological test surveys, and small samples of biologic fluids for qualitative or quantitative analyses.

Studies with Patient-Volunteers

1. A patient may be included as a volunteer in a research study unrelated to the disease or condition for which he is being treated if the study is not reasonably expected to interfere with the welfare of the patient or his treatment regimen and he otherwise satisfies the prerequisites of a volunteer.

2. When performing research with patient-volunteers, the investigator should obtain from the patient's physician an opinion that the patient may justifiably be included in the research project.

Studies with Nonpatient-Volunteers

In neuropsychopharmacologic research with volunteers, the attainment of scientific knowledge may be regarded as a primary goal. Research with volunteer subjects, i.e., mentally competent, fully informed adults, nevertheless imposes ethical responsibilities for the safety, dignity, and rights of these subjects.

Commentary

Many of the ethical problems dealt with in this Principle and in other Principles have been given thoughtful, detailed consideration in *Ethical Principles in the Conduct of Research with Human Participants*, published by the American Psychological Association (3).

PRINCIPLE 6: *ETHICAL RESPONSIBILITY – PHYSICAL AND MENTAL DISCOMFORT*

The scientific investigator has the obligation to minimize, to the extent possible, all undue physical and mental discomfort of the subject. When it appears that a research study may have resulted in undesirable consequences for the subject, the investigator shall make every reasonable attempt to detect them and to provide adequate follow-up treatment to remove, correct, or relieve those consequences.

Commentary

In scientific investigations of subjects involving physical and/or mental discomfort, the nature of the anticipated physical and/or mental discomfort should be explained to the subject in advance. Furthermore, the investigator should be reasonably certain, on the basis of existing knowledge, that the anticipated physical and/or mental discomfort will not have long-term adverse consequences for the nonpatient-volunteer.

PRINCIPLE 7: *ETHICAL CONSIDERATIONS IN EVALUATING POTENTIAL RESEARCH STUDY BENEFITS AND RISKS; RESEARCH PROCEDURES*

Patients

Research studies with patients shall be conducted only when the expectation of anticipated results will justify the experiment. At the time the research study is undertaken and throughout its performance, there should exist a scientific basis for a reasonable belief that the research may ultimately produce beneficial changes in the patient's clinical condition.

Patient-Volunteers and Nonpatient-Volunteers

1. Scientific gains expected from research studies with volunteers shall be weighed against the reasonably anticipated risks involved. At the time the research study is undertaken and throughout the performance, there should exist a scientific basis for a reasonable belief that the research study will ultimately produce scientific knowledge which will benefit patients in the future.

2. The scientific investigator shall not use a research procedure if it is likely to cause disabling or lasting harm to subjects or if the reasonably anticipated benefits to a patient are outweighed by reasonably foreseeable disadvantages.

Subjects of Limited Mental Capacity

1. Children may be subjects in a neuropsychopharmacologic research study when they need treatment and are reasonably expected to benefit from their participation in the study. They may also be included as "normal control" subjects in comparison studies. In general, research studies of drugs in children shall not be undertaken unless similar studies in adults have proved reasonably safe.

A drug that has been proved to be safe but ineffective in adults may be evaluated in children if there is a reasonable basis for expecting it to be effective in children. In some specific disorders which are unique to children, such as childhood autism, prior demonstration of drug efficacy in adults may be irrelevant. Research studies in these uniquely pediatric disorders are not foreclosed under this Principle because of the lack of such a disease process in adults.

2. A research study with subjects who are mentally incompetent or children involves additional considerations because of the limitations of the subjects or their inability to understand fully the procedures and implications of the research study and to communicate their feelings and responses to the investigator.

Inert Substances

The scientific investigator who proposes to use an "inert" substance (placebo) as part of the methodological requirement of a study shall examine carefully both the necessity and ethical considerations of the procedure as it relates to the specific illness or particular research problem (4). This approach shall be reviewed carefully by the Institutional Review Board or qualified review body.

The scientific investigator who proposes to use an "inert" substance as part of the research study shall carefully differentiate among patient groups in evaluating expected improvement against possible deterioration (4).

Commentary

Prior to the introduction of a neuropsychopharmacologic agent in man, studies of the agent in several different animal species shall have indicated the probability that a substantial risk of organ system injury will not result from its administration in man. However, in experimentation, it is impossible to predetermine the exact scope of the risks or benefits. This lack of precise foreknowledge of risks and benefits should be specified in the protocol and should be communicated to the subject, or in cases where informed consent cannot be obtained, to the person authorized to consent on his behalf. The existence of this uncertainty and honest realization of the limits of knowledge concerning the experiment should not in itself be the cause for abandoning the research.

The use of a placebo in severely ill patients, such as very disturbed and/or severely deteriorated chronic schizophrenic patients who present gross thought disorders and hallucinations, should be carefully reviewed by the investigator. It may be quite appropriate to use a placebo control group in evaluating treatment in conditions with a tendency toward spontaneous remission. Thirty to forty percent of patients diagnosed as acute schizophrenics may show moderate to marked improvement with placebo (5), while such improvement in very disturbed or severely deteriorated chronic schizophrenics is rare. In nonpsychotic conditions, such as anxiety and depression, the "superiority of standard existing drugs over placebo is of sufficiently modest extent to make the administration of placebo to some patients in a study justifiable, particularly if there are explicit provisions for removing from the study patients whose clinical condition worsened" (6).

Patients in any study, including those in which a placebo is being used, even under "blind" conditions, should be removed from the study at any clearly discernible sign of substantial worsening of their conditions and treated as expeditiously as possible.

PRINCIPLE 8: *INFORMED CONSENT*

The Requirements of Informed Consent

Research studies with human subjects require informed consent of the subjects. Where a subject lacks capacity to consent, the scientific investigator shall obtain the consent from a person authorized to give consent on behalf of the subject or shall take other legally appropriate action.

Informed consent as used in the context of these Principles is the agreement obtained from a subject (or from his authorized representative) to participate in a neuropsychopharmacologic research study. The basic elements of informed consent are:

1. An explanation of the procedures to be followed, including an identification of those that are experimental.

2. A description of the reasonably foreseeable attendant discomforts and risks and a statement of the uncertainty of the anticipated risks due to the inherent nature of the research process.

3. A description of the benefits that may be expected.

4. A disclosure of appropriate and available alternative procedures that might be advantageous for the subject.

5. An offer to answer any inquiries concerning the procedures.

6. A statement that information may be withheld from the subject in certain cases when the investigator believes that full disclosure may be detrimental to the subject or fatal to the study design *(providing,* however, that the Institutional Review Board has given *prior* approval to such withholding of information).

7. A disclosure of the probability that the subject may be given a placebo at some time during the course of the research study if placebo is to be utilized in the study.

8. An explanation of the probability that the subject may be placed in one or another treatment group and a definition of this probability in lay terms if randomization is a necessary part of the study design.

9. An instruction that consent may be withdrawn and participation in the study may be discontinued at any time.

10. An explanation that there is no penalty for not participating in or withdrawing from the study once the project has been initiated.

11. A statement that the investigator will inform his patient of any significant new information arising from the experiment or other ongoing experiments which might bear on the patient's choice to remain in the study (7).

12. A statement that the investigator shall provide a review of the nature and results of the study to those subjects who request such information.

Subjects Who Lack the Capacity to Consent

1. When a patient is mentally incompetent or too young to comprehend, informed consent must be obtained from one who is legally authorized to consent on behalf of the proposed subject. As the study progresses, the investigator also shall keep the person who consents on behalf of the subject informed of any major changes in the research protocol or significant side effects.

2. If a mentally incompetent or a retarded subject is capable of exercising some judgment concerning the nature of the research study and his participation in it, the investigator shall obtain the informed consent of the subject in addition to the person legally authorized to consent on his behalf.

3. When the subject is a child who has reached the age of some discretion, such as an adolescent, and the subject is otherwise mentally competent, the scientific researcher shall obtain the subject's informed consent in addition to the person legally authorized to consent on his behalf.

Consent of Prison Inmates and Other Especially Vulnerable Groups

1. With nonpatient-volunteers who are involuntarily institutionalized or subject to some legal restraint, the investigators should take special precautions to assure the subject the opportunity to obtain full information about the research study, including the right to refuse to participate or to withdraw from the study at any time without penalty.

2. When an investigator proposes to select as volunteer subjects individuals who are involuntarily institutionalized or subject to some legal restraint or whose personal circumstances are such that their need for volunteer compensation or course accreditation (students) may cloud their caution or judgment, the final approval concerning such a research study shall reside with the appropriate, qualified reviewing body.

Commentary

Consent of the subject is both a legal and ethical prerequisite. This *Statement of Principles* establishes the ethical requirements of consent, but takes no position on the legal sufficiency of the Principles.

The legal authority of a person to provide informed consent on behalf of one who lacks capacity may vary from state to state. Parental consent is usually required when children comprise the subject group in well-designed neuropsychopharmacologic experiments. However, the parent or court-appointed proxy has no legal or moral right to give consent for the child to participate in an experiment which has no specific etiologic, diagnostic, or therapeutic goals for the disease presented by the child, except in those cases where there are no "reasonably foreseeable risks" (8). With regard to persons who are mentally incompetent, some states may require informed consent from the closest living relative (9); some states may require consent by a legal guardian; and finally, some states may insist on approval from a court. The scientific investigator should make further inquiries to resolve any doubts he may have as to the appropriate person to give consent. This Principle does not contend that persons who may be vulnerable to undue influence must be automatically excluded as potential volunteers. Such decisions should be made by an appropriate Institutional Review Board on a protocol-by-protocol basis.

These Principles recognize the great difficulty that has surrounded the issue of informed consent. A further problem exists in subsequently proving, years later, that one did in fact secure informed consent. The use of forms detailing risks and benefits is presently the dominant means of dealing with this problem. An alternative procedure may involve the utilization of an individual not involved in the research study who would be present at the time consent is secured. Such an individual would assist the subject by explaining the risks and benefits to the subject and could certify for the purpose of documentation that informed consent had in fact been obtained. Utilization of such an individual would facilitate the explanation of risks and benefits in a manner appropriate for the subject, or person giving consent on his behalf, as well as providing subsequent proof of the occurrence of this procedure in the event of litigation.

A person who is incarcerated as a result of a criminal conviction should not be disqualified from being a volunteer in a neuropsychopharmacologic research study merely because he is a prisoner. Furthermore, a nonpatient-volunteer who is a prisoner should not be denied the opportunity to be exposed to a research study that undertakes an evaluation of an illness that may have been directly or indirectly associated with the prisoner's incarceration. For example, a prisoner with a history of heroin addiction that resulted in illegal activity and subsequent incarceration should have the opportunity to participate voluntarily in research studies of treatment with narcotic-blocking agents. If such a research endeavor were successful, the prisoner would then have gained a definite benefit from the particular experiment. However, the relative isolation of the prisoner from society and the inherently coercive environment of the prison imposes on the scientific investigator the additional obligation to take all practical measures to ascertain that the prisoner is truly a volunteer, that the prisoner understands that he is under no obligation to participate, and that the prisoner has full information about the study and its possible effects on him.

Careful consideration should be given to studies with residents of a poverty area whose need for paid volunteer fees may outweigh their caution or with college students who may participate in a drug research study if it is perceived as a requirement of a course or because of faculty pressure. Every volunteer is responding to some pressures; however, there is a difference between gross external pressures brought about, for example, by prison officials or teachers and internal pressures which are complex and vary among individuals. It may be difficult or impossible for the scientific investigator to be aware of and to evaluate complex internal pressures in a potential volunteer. The investigator should make special efforts to eliminate or decrease external pressures or reject volunteers who have been subjected to substantial external pressures.

PRINCIPLE 9: *SUBJECT'S RIGHT TO DECLINE OR WITHDRAW*

Right to Decline Participation and Right to Withdraw

The investigator shall respect the freedom of the individual subject or, in the case of those who lack capacity to consent, the person legally authorized to act on the patient's behalf to decline to participate in a research study or to discontinue participation at any time without penalty (10, 11).

Reviewing Body

The obligation to insure that the project protocol protects the subject's freedom to participate and withdraw is the responsibility of the reviewing body as well as of the individual investigator. The reviewing body shall determine whether or not the research procedures protect the subject from deceit or any type of undue influence.

Commentary

In studies with mentally competent individuals, the subject may withdraw from the research project at any time he chooses. However, patients unable to give informed consent pose particular problems (12). The scientific investigator assumes additional ethical responsibilities to the patient who, because of a lack of capacity, may not be able to make rational judgments concerning withdrawal from the research study. These additional responsibilities require exceptionally careful attention to a patient's attempted rejection of a particular treatment.

Regardless of the research subject's mental competency, the investigator may be uniquely able to anticipate adverse consequences from the continuation of an experiment. It is his responsibility to withdraw the patient from the study if such a situation appears imminent; this responsibility includes patients receiving either active drugs or placebo.

PRINCIPLE 10: *INFORMATION*

Confidentiality

The scientific investigator shall have responsibility for not improperly releasing information pertaining to subjects in the study. This responsibility includes not only information protected by law, which often does not apply to all subjects, but also information that affects the privacy and dignity of his subjects. When there is a likelihood that others may obtain access to such information derived from the research, the investigator, in obtaining informed consent, shall explain this possibility and his plans for maintaining confidentiality to the subject or, in the case of those lacking mental capacity, to the person who provides consent on behalf of the patient.

Explanation to Subjects

1. Information about foreseeable side effects should be given to the subject and/or the person who consented to the patient's treatment.

2. After the data are collected, the investigator shall provide a review of the nature and results of the study to those subjects who request such information. When scientific or humane values justify delaying or withholding information, the investigator incurs a special responsibility to take reasonable precautions that this action would not be expected to result in damaging consequences for the subject.

3. After termination of studies involving those who lack the capacity to consent, such as mentally incompetent persons and young children, the investigator shall reveal on request important and pertinent results to the person who provided consent for the patient.

PRINCIPLE 11: *ETHICAL OBLIGATIONS OF INVESTIGATOR FOR FOLLOW-UP TREATMENT OF THE PATIENT*

Responsibility of the Investigator to Communicate Research Results

The scientific investigator has the responsibility to inform the patient or the consenting person whether the research treatment has been effective or ineffective if the investigator believes that this information would be beneficial.

Responsibility for Follow-up Treatment for the Patient

The scientific investigator shall take reasonable steps to see that the patient is treated in the manner most appropriate to his needs. There steps may include the continuation of a research program if such a procedure is possible; if not, the best alternative should be sought.

REFERENCES

1. Federal Register-DHEW-PHS. Protection of human subjects: Policies and procedures. Vol. 39 (No. 105), May 30, 1974.
2. *The Institutional Guide to DHEW Policy on Protection of Human Subjects.* DHEW Pub. No. 72-102, Dec. 1, 1971.
3. Ad Hoc Committee on Ethical Standards in Psychological Research. *Ethical Principles in the Conduct of Research with Human Participants.* American Psychological Association, 1973.
4. Bishop, M.P., and Gallant, D.M. Observations of placebo response in chronic schizophrenic patients. *Arch. Gen. Psychiat.,* 14:497-503, 1966.
5. Gallant, D.M. *Summary Progress Report, 1974-1975.* PHS Grant No. MH03701-16.
6. FDA guidelines for psychotropic drugs. (Draft-June 1974). *Psychopharm. Bull.,* 4:7-28, 1975.
7. Fried, C. *Medical Experimentation: Personal Integrity and Social Policy.* New York: American Elsevier Publishing Co., 1974.
8. McCormick, R.A. Proxy consent in the experimentation situation. *Prospect. Biol. Med.,* 18(1):2-20, Autumn, 1974.
9. Attorney General of Louisiana. Opinion 74-1675, Nov. 14, 1974.
10. Nuremberg Code (Judgement on Experimentation without restriction). *United States v. Karl Brandt,* 1947. In: Katz, J. *Experimentation with Human Beings.* New York: Russell Sage Foundation, 1972, pp. 305-306.
11. Helsinki Code. *World Med. J.,* 11:281, 1964.
12. Gallant, D.M. Clinical and methodological considerations in psychotropic drug evaluation with schizophrenic patients. *Psychopharm. Bull.,* 6:4-12, 1970.

CHAPTER II

The History and Future of Litigation in Psychopharmacologic Research and Treatment

ALAN A. STONE

INTRODUCTION

The enterprise of psychopharmacologic research in the United States, particularly in its clinical aspects, currently faces a number of almost insuperable legal hurdles. These legal hurdles are the result of regulatory measures enacted by administrative and legislative bodies and of judicial decisions which have established precedents clearly or potentially applicable to psychopharmacologic research. This chapter will examine only the latter, the relevant case law (judicial decisions), which falls into three categories.

First, federal courts involved in the major right-to-treatment cases have included, in their lengthy decrees, stipulations about the right to refuse certain treatments and specifically the right to refuse experimental treatment.[1] Such specific provisions have been included by judges without any explicit or specific constitutional justification.[2] Nonetheless, litigating attorneys in other right-to-treatment cases will look to these provisions, and other judges may well accept them as precedents. Therefore, the research community must be aware of them and be prepared to react appropriately. Clinical psychopharmacologists doing research in any facility that falls under

---

[1] The right to refuse treatment has received increasing judicial protection, at least where extreme procedures are involved. See, for example, *Wyatt v. Aderholt* (1), *Wade v. Bethesda Hospital* (2), *Bell v. Wayne County General Hospital at Eloise* (3).

[2] See, for example, Judge Johnson's provisions (4, pp. 400-401). See also text pp. 22-23.

such a court decree risk criminal or civil contempt if they fail to comply.[3]

Second, a few courts, both state and federal, have found certain experimental procedures unconstitutional. This litigation involves what most psychiatrists consider extreme treatment modalities—i.e., experimental psychosurgery (5), myoneural blockade as behavior modification (6), and token economies (7,8) which begin under conditions deemed cruel and unusual punishment. It is a truism among lawyers that tough cases make bad law, but these are, in my view, easy cases that have made bad law. What has happened is that the case law and constitutional arguments built on these most extreme fact situations (e.g., experimental psychosurgery) are now being accepted and applied by judges, lawyers, and legal scholars to the regulation of much less intrusive research. These precedents, if applied, might mean that psychopharmacologic research could create liability in an institution's governing body or administration and among the research team for deprivation of the constitutional rights of the patient-subject.

Finally, there are tort actions or malpractice suits against physicians which are potentially applicable to research. Given the known side effects of psychotropic drugs, such as tardive dyskinesia, and the loose procedures attendant on research in the past, the paucity of appellate malpractice cases arising from research is extraordinary.

A BACKWARD GLANCE

Perhaps it will place the discussion that follows in perspective if I review one of the principal papers in the last *Psychopharmacology: A Review of Progress* in light of the legal constraints now applicable. I have chosen an overview paper by two doughty and well-known colleagues.

Cole and Davis (9) report on a survey of over 100 studies that, in evaluating the effectiveness of psychotropics, compared patients on psychotropics and patients on placebos. As Lehmann (10) notes in the same *Review of Progress,* the administration of a placebo to a patient who needs and would benefit from a known treatment is unethical and creates malpractice liability. It is my view that some of the placebo research documenting the effectiveness and limits of neuroleptics could have produced substantial malpractice liability even at the time it was conducted, and certainly would now.

For example, Cole and Davis (9, p. 1059) report a study by Gross et al.

---

[3] The major, right-to-refuse-treatment decrees have been spawned by a movement which calls for a re-examination of the legal foundations, consequences, and rights accompanying involuntarily committed residents in state mental hospitals. However, if the right to refuse treatment is to be implemented by the doctrine of informed consent— as the cases above indicate—then it would be hard not to apply the same rationales to any situation where voluntariness of and competence to give consent may be at issue.

(11) where 73 percent of the patients relapsed when active medication was withdrawn from psychotic patients being maintained in the community. If these patients had had substantial decompensations leading to hospitalization or to other significant pain and suffering, then they might well have had a good cause of action in a malpractice suit against those conducting the research, even if they had consented to participation. The well-known National Institute of Mental Health-Psychopharmacology Service Center (NIMH-PSC) collaborative study (12) from which much was learned about the treatment parameters of the phenothiazines creates the same malpractice liability since apparently many patients received inert placebos for a six-week period. Although Cole and Davis provide no information on whether the subjects in the various studies they surveyed were involuntarily confined at the time the research was undertaken, it is my impression that it was common practice to use committed patients as experimental subjects. Such practice today would, I believe, create serious liability and might well be the basis for a civil rights claim (13).

Ironically, a major legal text on civil commitment published in 1967, the same year as the last overview, presents the case history of a woman involuntarily confined to St. Elizabeth's Hospital in Washington, D.C., with an acute psychotic episode (14). This woman, with no semblance of a consent procedure, was placed in the control group of a neuropsychopharmacologic research project and received no drug treatment—this, despite the fact that she was obviously not dangerous and the reasons for confinement were based on the need for treatment. The authors of this casebook, certainly among the most eminent scholars in mental health law, make no mention of the constitutional or malpractice implications of these research practices. Such an omission would be unthinkable today.

Equally noteworthy is the fact that no appellate cases of any kind arose during the first fifteen years of neuropsychopharmacologic research. The current scene, therefore, speaks for the remarkable change in public and legal attitudes toward psychiatrists and medical experimentation generally. That same research today would surely produce a tidal wave of litigation.

The change in the attitude of physicians since the decade under review is also notable. Cole and Davis wrote from a posture of paternalism and "doctor knows best." For example, they comment on the value of fluphenazine enanthate as a "treatment of choice for acutely disturbed paranoid patients who are extremely reluctant to take medication" (9, p. 1062). If Cole and Davis had been as sensitive to the problems of informed consent then as they surely are now, that recommendation would have been much more carefully hedged. This is not to criticize my respected colleagues; rather, I wish to emphasize the dramatic changes that have occurred in our sensitivity to patients' rights since the *Review of Progress* was published in 1967. Thus, today, the administration of fluphenazine enanthate to a nonconsenting (reluctant), though acutely disturbed, paranoid patient creates possible legal and ethical problems that few of us dreamed of or were sensitive to ten years ago.

APPLICATIONS OF THE CONSTITUTION TO NEUROPSYCHOPHARMACOLOGIC RESEARCH

Right to Treatment

The most well known of the right-to-treatment cases is *Wyatt v. Stickney* (4), later *Wyatt v. Aderholt* (1), and still later *Wyatt v. Hardin*.[4] There, Judge Johnson, after holding hearings, formulated an order and decree holding, among other things, that:

> Patients shall have a right not to be subjected to experimental research without the express and informed consent of the patient, if the patient is able to give such consent, and of his guardian or next of kin, after opportunities for consultation with independent specialists and with legal counsel. Such proposed research shall first have been reviewed and approved by the institution's Human Rights Committee before such consent shall be sought. Prior to such approval, the Committee shall determine that such research complies with the principles of the Statement on the Use of Human Subjects for Research of the American Association on Mental Deficiency and with the principles for research involving human subjects required by the United States Department of Health, Education and Welfare for projects supported by that agency [4, pp. 401-402].

Judge Johnson here gave his judicial imprimatur both to the regulations of a federal agency[5] and to the principles developed by a quasi-private organization, the American Association on Mental Deficiency.[6] Further, he set up the terms of the consent procedures; namely, that the hospital must provide independent specialists and legal counsel to consult with the compe-

---

[4] By the time the three-judge panel of the Fifth Circuit Court of Appeals upheld the major holdings of *Wyatt v. Stickney,* Aderholt had been replaced by Hardin.

[5] The Department of Health, Education and Welfare (DHEW) has the power to impose conditions on dispensing of research grants. These rules reflect the importance of three principles: consideration of the rights and welfare of the subjects, acquisition by appropriate methods of informed consent, and determination of the risks and benefits of the investigation.

[6] Although the standards of the association do not carry the weight of legal formulations, they may impress any court because they are formulated by a group of intimately concerned professionals and lay persons who have weighed the pros and cons and developed the principles.

tent patient, and with his or her guardian or next of kin. It is interesting to note that there is no specific constitutional justification for these requirements; rather, the court, having taken upon itself the burden of trying to improve the quality of patient care, also takes on the responsibility of protecting patients from intrusive and experimental treatments. The difficulty of obtaining independent, capable, and willing specialists for consultation and the cost of hiring attorneys, of course, creates substantial burdens to research.

Careful readers of this judicial provision will note that it does not include a provision for obtaining consent when patients are incompetent. Thus, the provision created a situation in which no research could be done on incompetent patients even if it might benefit them.[7] Even more problematic, however, was a companion provision which, in the same manner, failed to provide a mechanism for incompetent patients to receive electroshock therapy (EST) or aversive therapy (4, pp. 400-401). It is still unclear to me whether this was judicial oversight or intentional. Judge Johnson has subsequently amended part, but not all, of these provisions. *Amici* did petition the judge specifically to allow aversive therapy of incompetent autistic children (15), presumably to control serious self-destructive or self-mutilating behavior, and the judge refused (see also Judge Johnson's denial as to autistic children [16]).

But the role of legal counsel in advising patients about participation in research presents the most interesting long-range question in Judge Johnson's decision. It is also relevant to much of the rest of this chapter, and therefore merits some discussion.

Lawyers have no obvious expertise or training in medical research. They must, and typically do, fall back on their traditional roles when they deal with the mentally ill. These traditional roles can be categorized, for my purposes, in two ways. The lawyer can simply function as a guardian *ad litem*—in many respects acting as a parent would, doing what he or she thinks best for the patient. Alternatively, the lawyer can function as an adversary, assuming that the proper role is to champion the patient against any intrusion by the proposed research, thus offering every possible legal argument against it, and forcing the researchers into a countering adversary posture. Whether any research at all will be possible in the future if lawyers adopt such an adversary posture remains to be seen. At the very least, I would assume that eventually every research project would be forced to hire a lawyer to deal with the adversary posture of the patient's lawyer.

However, whichever role is adopted by the attorney, it would seem to me

---

[7]Standard 29 of *Wyatt v. Stickney* (4, pp. 401-402) requires consent from the resident in *all* cases. Judge Johnson thus required the consent of the patient *and* a guardian or next of kin. "Incompetents" surely cannot meet the first requirement of self-assent.

that in the current climate and under a *Wyatt*-type decree, research that does not have a high likelihood of benefiting the particular patient is at an end in our state institutions. Even low-risk, nonbeneficial, but valuable research that does not serve the client's particular interest would probably be foreclosed by a lawyer who must look only to his client and give little or no weight to the value of the research to science or society. The specific reasons for this will become more obvious in the section that follows.

Restraints on Professional Practice

During the past decade there has been an enormous proliferation of mental health litigation aimed at institutional practice. Much of this litigation deals with the constitutional rights of involuntarily confined patients, but the decisions have had major implications for all inpatients, whatever their legal status.

The typical mental health litigation of the past decade was brought under 42 U.S.C. sec. 1983.[8] The statute reads:

> Every person who, under color of any statute, ordinance regulation, custom or usage of any state or territory, subjects or causes to be subjected any citizen of the United States to the deprivation of any rights, privileges, or immunities secured by the Constitution and laws shall be liable to the party injured in an action as law, suit in equity, or other proper proceeding for redress.

It is under this provisions of the Civil Rights Code that suits are brought for illegal arrest and detention, wire-tap invasions of privacy, etc. The scope of the sec. 1983 action has in the last ten years been widened to include the area of mental health law. Section 1983 actions can include injunctive and declaratory relief which asks the judge to declare the civil commitment statutes unconstitutional or to order the state to stop certain practices or change them.[9] Section 1983 actions have also, however, been pursued in the form of a personal damage action against mental health administrators and individual psychiatrists attached to state and private hospitals (19). The trend toward pressing for damages in civil rights litigation under sec. 1983 arrived with the landmark case of *Donaldson v. O'Connor* (20). The success of that case at the federal court level led litigating attorneys all over the country to crank out sec. 1983 actions against psychiatrists. Some, but not all, of these law suits ask for monetary damages.

---

[8] This statute will apparently form the basis for many more lawsuits based on current practice. See Caldwell and Brodie (17).

[9] For further discussion of complex issues regarding injunctive relief under other statutes, see Jacob (18).

Restraints on the Scope of Treatment

The bulk of the sec. 1983 civil rights litigation for damages deals with the scope of psychiatrists' lawful discretion to administer treatment, to order their patients' daily lives and living conditions, and to make decisions relative to the release of patients from a lawful commitment. Here it may not be obvious to psychiatrists that their actions are violating the rights of their patients. Every psychiatrist working in the public sector should know the *Donaldson v. O'Connor* standard articulated by the Supreme Court. A psychiatrist cannot continue to confine a patient who is not dangerous to himself or others and who can survive outside the hospital if he is not getting treatment (20, p. 576). Unfortunately, the Supreme Court did not define treatment or survival outside the hospital in any clear-cut way, but I think, at the very least, that they were saying that a psychiatrist who retains in involuntary custodial care a nondangerous patient who can survive outside the hospital is liable for violating that patient's civil rights.

Although, as yet, no federal court has recognized an absolute right of involuntary committed mental patients to refuse treatment, suits are now being litigated in that area (1-3). Regarding one Massachusetts hospital, a federal court issued a temporary restraining order that requires the hospital to allow patients to refuse treatment and that limits the use of seclusion. That order has apprarently led to an increase in assaults by unmedicated patients on other patients and on staff (21). Although the right to refuse treatment has not yet been clarified, courts have made it clear that the use of medication and seclusion for other than treatment reasons is a violation of patients' civil rights (22, 23).

The courts have also suggested that when medication is imposed on a Christian Scientist, whose religious beliefs are protected by the free exercise clause of the First Amendment, liability under a sec. 1983 action will result. *Winters v. Miller* (24) is such a case. However, despite the appellate decision, as of this writing, the case had not resulted in any damages being awarded, although Ms. Winters' lawyers intend to appeal still further.

All of these constitutional decisions which set new limitations on clinical practice will also have significant implications for clinical research in neuropsychopharmacology. Particularly significant will be the developments in the right to refuse treatment and the distinctions made between competent and incompetent refusals of treatment.

Proxy Consent

It is obvious that the appropriate subjects for neuropsychopharmacologic research are often mentally ill patients whose competence to give informed consent is in question. The traditional solution to this problem is to obtain informed consent from a close relative or guardian who then functions *in loco parentis* or as a "proxy." "Proxy consent" has become the subject of intense and prolonged debate among ethicists, philosophers, lawyers, and others because so many of the dilemmas of medical ethics seek resolution by developing some form of proxy consent. As we have already noted, Judge Johnson, without offering a legal or constitutional rationale, outlawed the use of proxy consent. Here I shall consider some of the articulated constitutional implications of proxy consent and other constitutional litigation particularly relevant to neuropsychopharmacologic research. *In this section, I am assuming that research is already being regulated under DHEW-type guidelines and the question is whether the Constitution mandates still more.* The major cases I shall discuss arose in exactly that context.

Parenthetically, it might be noted that sec. 1983 of the Civil Rights Act in some respects overlaps the traditional malpractice area or tort law. Presumably, patients might have sued their psychiatrists in state courts for malpractice rather than in federal courts for violation of their civil rights. Law reformers prefer the latter alternative because, on the one hand, it creates precedent, and, on the other hand, the federal tribunal and jury may be more sympathetic than the local state court. The result is, however, that psychiatrists may be vulnerable to two different kinds of legal liability for the same practice—e.g., placing a civilly committed patient in a neuropsychopharmacologic experiment without proper consent may lead either to a tort action or to a civil rights action. The latter may not be covered under the same medical liability insurance.[10] Indeed, it may in some states be impossible to indemnify psychiatrists against civil rights action. Furthermore, some insurers may not provide funds for legal defense.

Nielsen v. Regents: Paradigm for Proxy Consent

Several years ago, a group of researchers attempted to initiate a longitudinal study of allergic disease. Their experimental protocol involved two groups of children, one with high risk of developing allergy and a second low-risk control group. The protocol was approved by the Committee on Experimentation and the Human Rights Committee. A lawyer who was a member of the Human Rights Committee was, as he had been several times before, the lone objector to approval of the research. He decided to invoke a higher forum and brought a lawsuit in the Federal District Court, *Nielsen v. Regents* (25), seeking to prevent the use of children in the second control group for whom no benefit was anticipated.

He attacked the legitimacy of parental consent, alleging undue influence

---

[10] During personal involvement in the development of *Rogers v. Macht* (21) and other sec. 1983 litigation, insurers claimed that such actions and the legal defense to such actions were not provided by medical liability coverage.

in that, potentially, poor parents were to be paid $300 to absorb the atten-
dant expenses (baby sitters, travel, etc.). He also argued that the parents
drawn from the staff and student body of the university medical facilities
would be unduly influenced by their position vis-á-vis the senior staff sup-
porting and doing the research.

Commenting on this case, one law review note (26) asserts that these and
other factors as well suggest a conflict of interest between parent and child,
and that the child's interest in not being a subject of nonbeneficial experimentation should be protected by the Constitution. Specifically, the constitutional claim is that the child has either a right to privacy and/or bodily
integrity, and that that right cannot be gainsaid without due process of law,
and further, that the parents cannot be allowed to waive the due process
rights because of their conflicting interests and the alleged coercion of their
consent. Once one rejects the proxy consent of a parent, the consitutional
due process remedy to protect the right is, as one might expect, to provide
the child with an attorney and some form of evidential hearing consistent
with due process standards.

These kinds of constitutional arguments about parental consent for children are similar to those made in a recent landmark case where the Supreme
Court has granted cert. That case, *Bartley v. Kremens* (27), deals with the
parents' right to admit a child to a mental health facility. The federal court
below decided that the decision to admit a child to a mental health facility,
no matter how brief the stay and no matter how good the parental intention,
does involve a conflict of interest between parent and child (27). Further,
such hospitalization in a mental health facility does involve deprivation of
constitutionally protected rights. Therefore, the court erected due process
safeguards, including once again the appointment of an independent attorney
for the child within twenty-four hours of admission, a probable cause hearing
within seventy-two hours, and a full evidential hearing within fourteen days—
an evidential hearing at which the child might be present and the parents
subject to cross-examination.

The Attorney General of Pennsylvania, in a brief appealing the lower
federal court decision, argues that the autonomy of the family, recognized
both in common law and in a number of constitutional decisions (28-33),
should be the basis for rejecting this holding. The brief further argues that the
question of due process is never reached since a parental decision about a
child, which is a private action, and not a state action or state intervention
into the life of its citizens is at issue.

It is my view that the Attorney General's constitutional arguments, based
on their policy implications at least, have much to commend them. The
theory of *Nielsen* and *Bartley* is *first* that the child has constitutional rights,
and *second* that the parent cannot waive those rights because there is a pre-

sumed conflict of interest. It is the second aspect of the theory that I find troubling. It seems to me that traditional legal assumptions about conflicts of interest cannot readily be imposed on the parent-child relationship. From the legal perspective, family life is a constant conflict of interests: bedtime, boarding school, household chores, religious indoctrination are all parental decisions where there may be major conflict of interests and where one could argue that the child has constitutional rights worthy of protection. The law had traditionally avoided the pitfalls of intruding on family life by assuming an identity of interests between parent and child. Before assuming the opposite and imposing the constitutional paraphernalia of due process on parental decisions, it seems to me some clear threshold should be established for court intervention. One traditional standard and procedure for such legal intervention is child abuse, neglect, or abandonment, which are well-known legal concepts. That is the kind of clear standard I would apply as the threshold for legal intervention in parental decisions. Thus, I would argue that a parent should be allowed to waive constitutional rights and admit a child *under 12* to a mental health facility or enlist a child *under 12* in a research project, unless it can be demonstrated that there is probable cause to believe that the conditions of the hospital or the research are such as to constitute neglect, abuse, or abandonment. In my view, many institutions and some research have clearly fallen below that standard—e.g., the conditions at Willowbrook (23) in New York and the hepatitis research project conducted at that institution (34, pp. 1007-1010).

If we do not allow parents to abandon, abuse, or neglect their children in their homes, we should not allow them to place their children in institutions or experiments where such conditions exist. And if we allow parents to waive a child's right to privacy and sanctity of body in the home, parents should be able to waive those rights by enlisting children in a research project that has been approved by the Committee on Human Experimentation.

The approach I am suggesting would avoid the cumbersome due process resolution of these issues. It allows wide scope to parental authority and family autonomy, and it sets a familiar legal standard for court intervention. This solution will be unacceptable to some "child advocates" who are intent on building a wall of constitutional protection around children, without regard for the needs of the family as a whole and without recognizing that a wall that keeps others out can become a prison that locks the child in. A dramatic example of the intransigence of such child advocacy has been demonstrated in *Bartley v. Kremens* (27). The lower court ruling in favor of the child advocates cited the respite program for the mentally retarded as a clear conflict of interests between parent and child. The respite program allows parents who agree to keep their mentally retarded child at home to place the child in a facility for a week or two, allowing them a respite from the special demands of caring for such a child. The court fails even to recognize the value of such limited assistance to the family, or the counterproductive alternatives open to the family, such as abandoning the child entirely, if no respite is available.

Other Relevant Decisions

Courts have already gone beyond the kind of standards I suggest and have interfered with family autonomy in protecting the right of minors (usually over 12) to contraceptives and abortion. On the the subject of the minor's right to abortion, Justice Blackmun, writing for the majority, uses the following rhetoric: "Constitutional rights do not mature and come into being magically only when one attains the state-defined age of majority. Minors, as well as adults, are protected by the Constitution and possess constitutional rights." (35).

Despite this encompassing rhetoric, it is clear that these issues remain unresolved and that if Blackmun's principle were applied wherever applicable, parental authority and responsibility would be eviscerated of its traditional significance and meaning.

Nonetheless, the camel's nose is in the tent, and every constitutional argument that can be made by self-appointed child advocates applies *a fortiori* to the adult mentally disabled. If there is a potential conflict between parent and child as to participation in nonbeneficial research, surely there is such a conflict between spouses. If children are entitled to due process in that context, then surely adults are. If we pursue these arguments, we begin to recognize the possible constitutional problems of obtaining proxy consent to do research when patient-subjects are themselves not competent to consent.

The author of the law review note on *Nielsen v. Regents* concluded that "the most acceptable solution would be to discontinue all nonbeneficial research on children" (26, pp. 1173-1175). Failing that result, the author calls for judicial review of any child's participation in nonbeneficial research. During such judicial hearings, the traditional presumption that there is an identity of interests between parent and child is to be discarded.

The Luddite mentality of much of the legal writing on medical research is exemplified in the Draconian recommendation to "discontinue all nonbeneficial research on children" (26, pp. 1173-1175). But the callous and overreaching use of children and of the mentally disabled in research by prestigious physicians and institutions in the past is painful evidence of the opposite extreme having prevailed in medicine. Given these polar extremes, is a sensible answer to be found through constitutional litigation? The answer, it seems to me, depends on what kind of constitutional litigation, applied to what kind of research.

Cruel and Unusual Punishment

I have already indicated that the due process solution seems to be inappropriate since it involves the appointment of attorneys and the judicial review of the participation of each incompetent patient-subject. The cost in money, time, and energy of this "due process solution" would alone be sufficient to prevent most research, particularly since it is in addition to institutional review, an already cumbersome procedure. However, several cases have been litigated in which a different constitutional argument has been made; namely, that the experimental research itself constituted cruel and unusual punishment, and thus violated the Eighth Amendment. *Mackey v. Procunier* (36) is a case in point. There the Ninth Circuit Court of Appeals held that experimentation in aversive therapy at Vacaville in California that utilized succinylcholine raised "serious constitutional questions respecting cruel and unusual punishment."

Another case, *Knecht v. Gillman* (37), at the Iowa Security Medical Facility, involved aversive conditioning with apomorphine without informed consent. Again, the Eighth Amendment was invoked by the court.

These decisions, though their exact constitutional significance is unclear, stand for the proposition that courts can bar certain kinds of intrusive research on prisoners and mentally disabled patients on constitutional grounds of cruel and unusual punishment. This application of the Constitution quite sensibly looks to the humane treatment of the patient-subjects, rather than erecting elaborate procedural hurdles to research even where risk is absent or minimal. At the constitutional level, the Eighth Amendment approach is analogous to the threshold standard of child abuse, neglect, or abandonment, which I put forward earlier.

The Kaimowitz Decision

The ultimate constitutional constraints on research with psychiatric patients have been articulated by the *Kaimowitz* court which dealt with psychosurgery (5). This case arose after the various relevant committees had approved a research project to compare the effects of drug intervention (cryptoterone acetate) and amygdallotomy on uncontrollable aggression. The potential patient, John Doe, chose to submit to surgery rather than anti-androgen therapy. The *Kaimowitz* court focused on the psychosurgery and therefore dealt with two questions:

> First, after failure of established therapies, may an adult or a legally appointed guardian, if the adult is involuntarily detained at a facility within the jurisdiction of the State Department of Mental Health, give legally adequate consent to an innovative or experimental surgical procedure on the brain, if there is demonstrable physical abnormality of the brain, and

the procedure is designed to ameliorate behavior which is either personally tormenting to the patient, or so profoundly disruptive that the patient cannot safely live, or live with others?

Second, if the answer to the above is yes, then is it legal in this state to undertake an innovative or experimental surgical procedure on the brain of an adult who is involuntarily detained at a facility within the jurisdiction of the State Department of Health if there is demonstrable physical abnormality of the brain, and the procedure is designed to ameliorate behavior which is either personally tormenting to the patient, or so profoundly disruptive that the patient cannot safely live, or live with others? [5, p. 5].

After a long and somewhat ambiguous constitutional and policy argument, the court concluded that John Doe, the potential experimental patient, was unable to give consent to psychosurgery. They further concluded that "the guardian or parent cannot do that which the patient, absent a guardian, would be legally unable to do" (5, p. 16).

After concluding that it was impossible in this situation to obtain consent to participate in experimental psychosurgery either from the patient or from the proxy consenter, the *Kaimowitz* court turned to constitutional issues. Their first consideration was over the application of the First Amendment.

The First Amendment Argument and Research

"A person's mental processes, communication of ideas, the generation of ideas, come within the ambit of the First Amendment" (5, p. 19). Since the brain is responsible for generating ideas, brain surgery raises First Amendment questions. Therefore, to allow experimental psychosurgery under these circumstances is "to condone State action in violation of basic First Amendment rights of such patients, because impairing the power to generate ideas inhibits the full dissemination of ideas" (5, p. 22).

The *Kaimowitz* court noted that the counsel for John Doe had argued persuasively that the Eighth Amendment was applicable to this case. The *Kaimowitz* court felt it was unnecessary to reach that question because of the other legal and constitutional reasons "for holding that the involuntarily detained mental patient may not give an informed and valid consent to experimental psychosurgery" (5, pp. 24-25).

The kinds of First Amendment constitutional arguments made in *Kaimowitz* have been most fully developed by Shapiro (38). Shapiro has laid the groundwork for an encompassing theory that all involuntary somatic therapies, including psychoactive drugs, by affecting the mind, affect the capacity to generate ideas and, therefore, all such treatments, be they experimental or not, raise First Amendment questions. As I understand his argument, any time anyone affects the mind or brain of another person without that other person's consent, there is an infringement of constitutional rights. Shapiro's arguments cast a shadow not only on research on neuropsychopharmacology, but on much of ongoing neuropsychopharmacologic treatment as well. These constitutional issues are now all part of the ongoing debate on the right to refuse treatment. The resolution of that debate will have the utmost significance for clinical research in neuropsychopharmacology.

The Meaning of Consent

The case law I have thus far discussed can be usefully re-examined from a somewhat different perspective. Informed consent and proxy consent are central to *Kaimowitz* and *Nielsen,* but the meaning and significance of these concepts remain unclear.

The *Kaimowitz* court's reasoning has baffled and frightened some legal commentators because it can be read as suggesting that prisoners cannot give their informed consent to anything. Similarly, if the argument in *Nielsen* is correct, that a parent should not be able to consent to nonbeneficial research on his or her child, why should the parent be allowed to consent to beneficial research which entails greater pain, risk, or stigma than that produced by available treatment methods?

The point is that the closer one looks at informed consent and proxy consent, the more one becomes convinced that they are both slippery slopes, leading to the conclusion that no one is ever truly informed and that no one is entitled to be a proxy consenter. The empirical evidence all confirms the great difficulty of providing informed consent for medical procedures. On the other hand, decisions like *Kaimowitz* suggest that the real concern was judicial fear of psychosurgery and not judicial concern about informed consent or proxy consent. I have increasingly become convinced that informed consent is a legal fiction which in reality serves three social policy goals that have no relation to individual autonomy or freedom of choice. First, as we have seen, informed consent can be used as a procedural device to block research and treatment that is disfavored by some pressure group. This use of informed consent has become blatantly obvious in other contexts. For example, the Utah legislature, which objected to the Supreme Court decision on abortion (39), set up a statutory requirement for informed consent that is potentially guilt-inspiring and humiliating to the pregnant woman who wants an abortion (40). California's legislature adopted a similar approach attempting to restrain EST through, among other things, the consent procedure (41).

These are overt examples of what happens covertly in other instances where, behind the smokescreen of informed consent, the real battle is being waged over what kind of research and treatment our society will accept.

The second social policy objective behind the courts' expansion of informed consent is to permit causes of action and compensation for plaintiffs who suffer as the result of some adversity of medical treatment. Although it can be argued that the policy goals, cited by courts as having inspired the expansion of informed consent, are aimed at promoting the opportunity for patients to make informed decision about their lives, the empirical evidence suggests the futility of such an objective (see generally: Ingelfinger [42] ; see also Barber et al. [43] and Gray [44]).

The third social policy is related to the second—namely, the demystification of the medical profession and the radical transformation of the doctor-patient relationship from one defined by status to one defined by contract (45). Surely the proliferation of standard informed-consent forms devised by lawyers so that doctors can meet the new legal requirements of informed consent has added little to patient autonomy or independence. The patient must now cope with not only the jargon of medical technology, but also the jargon of legal pseudotechnology. It is, of course, possible to prepare an informed-consent form written so that the ordinary lay person can understand the various medical implications of a proposed course of treatment. Indeed, I was asked to assist in the preparation of such a form to be used with neuroleptics. I find it hard to believe that a majority of patients reading the form proposed would agree to treatment, particularly after they read the description of tardive dyskinesia written in plain English: "I understand that treatment with (neuroleptic drugs) may lead to my developing movements of my mouth/tongue/face/body which are involuntary and may be irreversible. Little is known about the cause of these movements or their treatment."

It may well be that a radical reduction in the prescription of neuroleptics would be a good thing. Perhaps the medical profession has been imposing risk-benefit ratios which patients would find unacceptable. However, striking the optimal balance will not be achieved by frightening patients.

Unfortunately, medicine does have skeletons in the closet, and that reality, together with the new mood of consumer protection, leads to an increasing level of suspicion among reformers. Since it is the reformers who take the initiative in litigation and legislation, one can expect that the changing legal doctrine of informed consent will reflect an attitude of distrust of medical authority.

Summary

This section has attempted to suggest how First Amendment, Eighth Amendment, and due process constitutional arguments might conceivably apply to clinical research in neuropsychopharmacology. I have expressed the view that the Eighth Amendment approach, analogous to the child-abuse approach, is the appropriate parameter if there is to be constitutional intervention in addition to Human Rights Committee regulation of research. The approach suggested avoids erecting cumbersome procedural impediments that are beyond the capacity of courts already overburdened and overextended.

It should again be emphasized that I have rejected case-by-case judicial review and due process safeguards on the basis that they are in addition to the kind of regulation mandated by DHEW and other controlling agencies. As to the First Amendment approach advocated by Shapiro (36), it gathers into its net not only research, but, in addition, so many medical and nonmedical activities that it falls under the maxim that by including everything, it includes nothing.

TRADITIONAL MALPRACTICE LAW AS IT APPLIES TO NEUROPSYCHOPHARMACOLOGIC RESEARCH

The problems of consent have long been central to the tort law, and I turn now to that more traditional case law to emphasize, once again, the absence of decisions that deal directly with neuropsychopharmacologic research.

The tort law suggests that unless the patient consents or the doctor acts in an emergency, then medical treatment may be a battery (46, 47). This is theoretically true even if the treatment is excellent and the physician's therapeutic motives above question.[11] *A fortiori,* the physician who experiments on a patient without consent is liable for battery. As I have already indicated, however, the problem that is central to the group of patients for whom neuropsychopharmacologic treatment is intended is the competency of consent.

The traditional tort law has usually allowed proxy consent by the parents, guardian, or nearest relative for the incompetent patient. The case law, however, assumes that medical treatment is in the patient's best interest (49)—an assumption that obviously does not necessarily apply to research that is either nonbeneficial or where the risk-to-benefit ratio is higher than in other available treatment. The recent kidney donor cases (50-52), which are familiar to many physicians, squarely raise this issue. The parents may be asked to consent to a child's donation of a kidney to a sibling. The surgeon in these cases has to decide whether such proxy consent is valid and will protect him from liability. Increasingly, physicians and hospitals are turning to the courts to obtain a judicial imprimatur where, as in the kidney donor cases, the procedure is not in the donor's best interest. It has been argued that the psychological benefit of forestalling the death of a sibling is greater than the

---

[11]*Mohr v. Williams* (48), for example, makes it clear that the injury is to dignity.

physical and psychological risks of anesthesia, nephrectomy, and life with one kidney for the donor (50, pp. 390-391).

Whether or not one agrees with the substantive merit of such weighing and balancing of altruistic psychological benefits, these do not seem to me the kind of benefits contemplated in the case law.[12] One can at least imagine a society in which the obligations of family were so prized that the law and tradition would require a brother to save his brother, if not by donating a kidney, then at least by donating bone marrow. But in our society, oriented to individual rights and erosive of family obligation, there are no such duties recognized in law. Therefore, the courts must either rationalize that it is in the child's best interest to sacrifice his kidney or bone marrow, or not authorize the procedure. (See, for example, *Strunk v. Strunk* [55], but see also *Hart v. Brown* [50 pp. 390-391] where the court allowed transplant simply because the twin donor's kidney had greatest likelihood of success.)

Since, in my view, the court has no clear legal or moral guidelines for defining the "best interest" in this context, what has happened is that the judge imposes his judgments rather than the parents. The judge has become in this system the proxy consenter.

The ethical guidelines for neuropsychopharmacologic research contain an interesting moral principle relevant to this discussion: "Scientific research does not exist in a vacuum. It should be emphasized that all persons living in society have a moral responsibility to participate in efforts to promote and contribute to the present and future welfare of that society. Research is one of these obligations" (56). This "inherent obligation" to make an altruistic contribution is exactly the element that is lacking in the law when it seeks to resolve these questions.

The legal conception of informed consent has recently undergone revision in some states (57-60). The old standard was to tell the patient what other physicians told the patient (61, 62). The new standard is to tell the patient what a reasonable person would want to know (57-60). This latter standard is obviously both more comprehensive and more difficult for the guild of physicians to determine. The new standard reflects the reformist orientation already described. It is my view that whatever the malpractice standard is for treatment, the standard for research must be even more exacting.

The pattern of future tort litigation on research will follow the pattern of future malpractice litigation. It is my impression that psychiatrists and others prescribing neuroleptics have failed to obtain appropriate consent forms

---

[12]The courts (50-52) have succumbed to an expansive concept of benefit. Under a strict interpretation of benefit, altruism or avoidance of possible psychological harm should not qualify. *In accord: In re Richardson* (53), slip opinion, p. 5. *Contra:* Skegg (54).

where they have obtained them at all. Although it may be possible to rationalize this failure under the older consent standard, it is, in my view, impossible to justify the failure to inform patients about the risks of tardive dyskinesia under the new standard.

Whatever standard is applicable in a given jurisdiction, there is already reason to anticipate a wave of malpractice litigation against physicians prescribing neuroleptics because of tardive dyskinesia.[13] Failure of physicians to inform patients of the possibility of tardive dyskinesia will surely be an element in these lawsuits. I personally have no doubt about the outcome, and surely the disfigurement of tardive dyskinesia will lead juries to grant large awards. Research with new neuroleptic drugs obviously must anticipate the possibility of such litigation.

There may well be other grounds for negligence of interest to those doing neuropsychopharmacologic research. For example, it is possible that prescription of neuroleptics to patients whose condition does not justify the risks of neuroleptics will be considered negligence.[14] Thus, the large-scale treatment of the mentally retarded, of prisoners, and of other patient populations without psychotic disorder for purposes of behavior control will produce a significant number of cases of tardive dyskinesia and malpractice litigation. Such prescription of neuroleptics, even with informed consent, may in itself be negligent. Neuropsychopharmacologic research that attempts to apply neuroleptics to new conditions must be aware that a patient or proxy may not be able to give informed consent to a treatment that has inappropriate risks, given the condition.[15]

Finally, many physicians prescribing neuroleptics are unaware of the appropriate diagnostic examinations for detecting the onset of tardive dyskinesia or of the fact that larger dosages will mask the onset. Thus, they may be negligent in failing to detect the onset of symptoms when, arguably, the possibility of reversibility and minimization of tardive dyskinesia is greater. Obviously those doing neuropsychopharmacologic research should be held to the highest standard of competence in this regard.

These are by no means the only grounds for tort liability that might attach to neuropsychopharmacologic treatment and research, but they are meant to indicate the serious pitfalls that will constrain the next decade of progress in neuropsychopharmacologic research.

---

[13]Where patients were not informed of the possible and significant side effects of treatments courts have found doctors liable (63-65).

[14]See Prosser (46, Secs. 9, 32) for rationales as to why battery or negligence may form a basis for liability.

[15]See *Kaimowitz* (5) slip opinion that stresses the relatively unproven appropriateness of a "treatment" modality as a basis for a finding of incompetency to give consent.

CONCLUSION AND RECOMMENDATION

During the summer of 1976, it became apparent that the distribution of swine flu vaccine would not be possible unless the pharmaceutical houses could obtain government indemnification of their liability against tort claims. The reason for the difficulty in obtaining private indemnification arises from the developments of tort law similar to those I have touched on. It may well be that if neuropsychopharmacologic research is to continue in this country, it too will require some form of governmental indemnification. Obviously, the United States can take no ethical satisfaction if litigation and regulation prevents research on American citizens, while we use new drugs developed on the citizens of other nations. We will simply have subjected citizens of other countries to yet another form of exploitation and colonization.

COMMENTARIES

MR. SCOTT: Dr. Stone notes that recent litigation has raised a number of important questions for psychopharmacologic research and treatment. Cases brought to correct grossly substandard conditions in mental health and retardation facilities and to stop or regulate hazardous and abusive practices have led to the recognition of patients' rights to which neither lawyers nor mental health professionals, as Dr. Stone points out, had previously been sensitive. These newly recognized rights create some rather obvious needs for a review of the manner in which treatment is administered or imposed and research is conducted. In some instances, difficult problems are arising which do not readily lend themselves to solutions that satisfy all legitimate interests.

Psychopharmacologists and mental health professionals are not unique in having to face new difficulties and to deal with criticisms from previously unheard-from quarters. Throughout our society, matters traditionally considered the relatively exclusive domain of particular institutions are being opened to review by and accountability to "outside" groups. Thus the societal, moral, and ethical implications of the activities of corporations, schools, prisons, and the legal and medical professions, to name just a few, have been brought under public scrutiny; and the practices and precepts of these entities have been examined and challenged by ethicists, civil rights and consumer groups, environmentalists, legislatures, and, of course, the courts. Psychopharmacology cannot expect to be exempt. It is an important field of endeavor having significant consequences for millions of Americans. Its activities ought to be of great interest and concern to the public. Accordingly, I believe that it will have to deal with other segments of society having legitimate concerns about the ethical, legal, moral, and societal implications of psychopharmacologic research and treatment.

The opening up of isolated or insulated enterprises can, however, precipitate turmoil and confusion. And the end results of more open, more complex decision-making processes can be mixed blessings.

In my view, however, major mental health law developments, even those arising out of so chancey an undertaking as litigation, have been occurring in a remarkably logical and thoughtful fashion. Whatever disadvantageous ramifications there have been do not, I believe, even approach the point of bringing the value of the patients' advocacy movement into question. An important contributing factor to this relative lack of major detriments has been the active participation of progressive mental health professionals and their national associations and of patients and consumer groups in many of the leading cases. The American Psychiatric Association, American Psychological Association, American Association on Mental Deficiency, National Association for Mental Health, and other groups have contributed as *amici curiae* (friends of the court) in several cases.[16] Also, when such groups have not formally been involved, their leadership has often been consulted, and major suits are typically planned in advance with prominent leaders in the fields of mental health and retardation.

At the present time, litigation and potential litigation is arising in areas of increasingly direct concern to the American College of Neuropsychopharmacology. The College itself and leaders in this field may be consulted or asked to participate in lawsuits or legislative efforts that raise hard questions and require carefully considered, sophisticated solutions. There will be a premium on interdisciplinary collaboration in the interest of the further orderly changes needed to adjust current practices to emerging rights.

I am therefore concerned that Dr. Stone's paper, by virtue of its tone and emphasis and its unremittingly harsh criticisms of the legal advocates of the interests of child and adult mentally disabled patients, may serve to create undue animosity and distrust. Litigation has not brought psychopharmacologic research and treatment to a halt. In fact, very few cases have directly involved any aspect of psychopharmacology in a way that could be characterized as impeding arguably legitimate treatment and research to any significant extent. The actual picture is not that of constitutional litigation having hobbled sound clinical practice and good research, but that of doubts and

---

[16] For example, the American Psychological Association, American Orthopsychiatric Association, American Association on Mental Deficiency, and National Association for Mental Health participated as *amici* at both the trial and appellate levels in *Wyatt v. Stickney* (66). The American Psychiatric Association was an *amicus* at the appellate level and argued in favor of affirmance.

questions having arisen as to the potential impact of constitutional litigation. These doubts and questions can best be addressed and resolved through open discourse in which we each voice our concerns, listen to each other and to other interested groups, and strive to reach optimal solutions.

Turning to the content of Dr. Stone's paper, I should first summarize the substantive thrust of his paper with regard to constitutional issues. He contends that the courts should not be concerned with research programs unless (a) in the case of a child, there is reason to believe that child abuse, abandonment, or neglect exists, or (b) in the case of an adult, the patient is being subjected to cruel and unusual punishment. Thus, as long as "DHEW-type guidelines" are followed, he argues that courts should not consider constitutional challenges. Specifically, he takes the position that the courts should not impose additional procedural due process requirements, nor should they set standards regarding the quality of the patient-subject's consent.

In criticizing procedural due process requirements, he asserts that they would be too costly and that, if they involved the provision of counsel to prospective subjects, much valuable research would be precluded. With regard to the concept of informed consent, he portrays it as a "legal fiction" that serves purposes not related "to individual autonomy or freedom of choice."[17]

Thus, in the interest of facilitating unhampered research, Dr. Stone presents a case for limiting constitutionally based judicial intervention. In taking this approach, I think that he has missed the opportunity to begin working with leaders in psychopharmacologic treatment and research on acceptable solutions to the perceived difficulties recent litigation poses for them.

With regard to some of the specifics of Dr. Stone's contentions, first it seems rather unlikely to me that the courts will ultimately hold that the only constitutional rights that mentally disabled patients and psychiatric research subjects have with respect to treatment are freedom from child abuse and from cruel and unusual punishment, and that even with respect to these

---

[17]While the text of my commentary does not take issue with Dr. Stone's total disparagement of the role of informed consent, I must note my disagreement. His assertion that *Kaimowitz v. Department of Mental Health of the State of Michigan* (15) may be read as suggesting that prisoners cannot give their consent to anything overlooks the fact that the court was careful to note that the unattainable standard of consent it required for experimental psychosurgery would not apply to less hazardous or intrusive procedures. (See slip opinion at pp. 21-22.) More importantly, I believe that the notion of informed consent has an extremely important role to play in the future. It is a key concept in imparting an active, responsible role to patients in treatment decision making. If some treatment facilities demean this role by reducing informed consent to mere forms reminiscent of aluminum-siding contracts, as Dr. Stone suggests, there must be ways to overcome such ploys.

minimal rights the Constitution requires no procedural due process safe-guards. Fairly extensive legal precedents are establishing a clear trend toward recognizing that the constitutional right to privacy and the First Amendment include protection of the individual's autonomous control over his or her own mental and emotional processes.[18] These state and lower federal court decisions are bolstered by United States Supreme Court rulings. For example, *Stanley v. Georgia* (70):

> Our whole constitutional heritage rebels at the thought of giving government the power to control men's minds . . . Whatever the power of the state to control dissemination of ideas inimical to public morality, it cannot constitutionally premise legislation on the desirability of controlling a person's private thoughts.

Because the nonconsensual administration of psychotropic drugs impinges on one's autonomous control, it may be viewed as an infringement on constitutionally protected rights. The notion that at least some forms of mental health treatment are so intrusive, i.e., capable of effecting substantial changes in mental activity without the individual's cooperation, or so hazardous that their administration may infringe on constitutionally protected freedom shows marked signs of vitality.[19]

It is important to note, however, that the determination that a particular action infringes on a constitutionally protected right does not necessarily mean it is not permissible (73). Rather, that determination usually brings into play certain other constitutional principles by which the permissibility of the action may be measured. First, most constitutional rights can be waived; and, if the individual is capable of giving competent, informed, and voluntary consent, his consent will ordinarily be accepted as a waiver of the constitutional rights at issue (74, 75). Second, if the individual is incapable of giving consent or refuses to give it, the action might be justified as necessary to achieve a legitimate state interest of sufficient importance to outweigh the infringement (76, 77). Third, infringements of privacy and First Amendment rights must be no greater than is necessary to achieve the relevant state interest (78, 79). Application of this principle—the "least

---

[18] See *Scott v. Plante* (67), *Mackey v. Procunier* (6), *Winters v. Miller* (24)—decided primarily on grounds of freedom of religion, *Price v. Sheppard* (68)—requiring court approval for the nonconsensual administration of "the more intrusive forms of treatment," *Kamowitz* (5). See also *Wyatt v. Hardin* (69).

[19] See the cases cited in fn. 18. These cases reverse a trend in earlier cases suggesting that treatment should be administered over possibly competent objection. See *Whitree v. State* (71) and *Nason v. Superintendent of Bridgewater State Hospital* (72).

drastic means" test—in individual treatment situations may result in a constitutional preference for the use of the least intrusive and least hazardous of available treatments of equivalent efficacy (80, 81).

Finally, under procedural due process principles, the courts generally insist on procedural safeguards to assure that these constitutional principles are observed and that the individual has the opportunity to assert any opposition he may have to the proposed infringement (e.g., *Scott v. Plante* [67, p. 946]; *Knecht v. Gillman* [37]—specifying safeguards to ensure the voluntariness of consent to an aversive conditioning program). How much "process" is "due" in any given situation, however, varies according to the nature of the societal and individual interests at stake (82, 83). For example, the Supreme Court has held that before a child can be suspended from school for ten days or less, he is entitled only to notice as to what he is accused of, an explanation of the evidence, and a chance "to present his side of the story" (84). But, before a child may be adjudicated as a juvenile delinquent, he is entitled to representation by defense counsel and to a judicial hearing in which the rules of evidence and most procedural rights afforded criminal defendants are observed (85). A similar flexibility can be expected in the mental health area.

But one should also expect that the courts will note the special vulnerabilities and handicaps of mentally disabled patients and, therefore, require or approve of procedural safeguards that provide special protection (86). When voluntariness and competence are in doubt, e.g., in the cases of involuntary and institutionalized patients, and when the proposed technique is highly intrusive or hazardous, required procedures may include the appointment of counsel and the conduct of administrative or judicial review (67, 69).

In connection with the role of counsel in such matters, I feel constrained to take particular issue with Dr. Stone. He asserts that, lacking "expertise or training in medical research," lawyers "must . . . fall back on their traditional roles," which he characterizes as either that of a "guardian *ad litem*" who does "what he or she thinks best for the patient" or that of "an adversary [who] champion[s] the patient against any intrusion." Dr. Stone here overlooks some of the more significant responsibilities and skills of lawyers. Perhaps the most striking omissions are those of advisor and of advocate of the client's express desires. After painstaking and, I would hope, patient and sensitive consultation involving the advice of an appropriately qualified, independent mental health professional, the client may well express the desire to participate in the proposed research or treatment. In that event, the attorney should respect the client's wishes, but he may still act to ensure that the hazards are minimized and that the client's interests are otherwise protected. Other significant roles for the lawyer in this context are to help the client resist coercive influences, to explore other alternatives, and to attempt to negotiate compromise solutions that might be acceptable to both the treatment staff and the client.

There is considerable evidence that lawyers can and do play such constructive roles in the mental health field (87, 88).[20] I would, however, acknowledge that there are some who appear so mystified by psychiatric expertise that they fail to serve as true advocates (88, 90). But I view that phenomenon as a transient problem that will most likely right itself as the bar awakens to its responsibilities to the mentally disabled.

The involvement of lawyers in those areas of psychopharmacologic research and treatment where the needs for procedural protections are greatest is not the fearsome spectre that some might imagine. Surely it will add to the costs, but there will be clear benefits in the form of enhancement of the informed and voluntary quality of consent of those who do participate, greater protection of the individual from real or apparent coercive pressures, and a more careful observation of individuals' legal rights. I would also venture to speculate that research as a whole may be improved through exposure to the scrutiny of lawyers who, if their clients are to be included in experimental treatment programs, will seek assurance that the programs actually have scientific merit.[21]

My own advice to those involved in psychopharmacologic research and treatment is to heed the import of recent litigation in this area. The administration of physically and psychically intrusive or hazardous treatments when the voluntary and informed quality of the patient's or subject's consent is not assured does raise important constitutional issues founded on principles of privacy and personal autonomy. Procedures that are responsive to these issues need to be fashioned. Before you encounter litigation, and even in the context of some cases, you will have the opportunity to help develop accommodations between treatment and research objectives and the personal freedom of patients and subjects. Many acceptable accommodations may be possible through strengthening existing review mechanisms. For example, increasing the institutional independence of review boards and committees and making arrangements for the provision of independent legal advocates and mental health consultants for research subjects may resolve some po-

---

[20] For a very interesting portrayal of the record of an interdisciplinary advocacy service in representing children in commitment proceedings, see the Brief of Department of the Public Advocate (89).

[21] A social worker on the staff of the Mental Health Law Project recently made a review of 63 studies of phenothiazine use on mentally retarded persons. She found that 76 percent failed to meet even half of the six basic criteria for satisfactory drug studies with children set forth in Sprague and Werry (91) and Marker (92). See also Marholin and Philips (93) who analyze eight of the eleven best studies on chlorpromazine and find "a consistent set of methodological flaws in each . . ."

tential problems.[22] Also, your participation in the design of legislative measures intended to implement newly recognized rights of mentally disabled patients could enhance the practicality and efficacy of such laws from your viewpoint and that of your patients.

Both the bar and the mental health professions are learning that they owe more and greater duties to mentally disabled patients than they previously acknowledged. Neither group can afford to ignore or minimize these responsibilities. And each needs the cooperation and advice of the other in order to make its own best contribution to the needs of the mentally disabled.

MS. HOLDER: To Dr. Stone's discussion of some major issues in research with patients who may be considered incompetent, I would like to add only some views on the nature of informed consent in general and proxy consent on behalf of children in particular. Dr. Stone gives the impression that he feels that the recent legal developments in these areas present a serious problem for both the researcher and the practitioner. While I agree with his analysis of the significance of most of the other legal issues, such as the effect of the Civil Rights Act on the rights of mentally disabled patients (although I trust his discussion makes clear to those of you who are not lawyers that this Act applies only to patients in public institutions and does not affect patients committed to private hospitals), I do believe that recent developments in the law regarding informed consent are less threatening to the future of biomedical research than he indicates. Our differences are not primarily related to the current state of the law, although I do take issue with his analysis of the recent Supreme Court decision on a minor's right to consent to an abortion. For the most part, we agree what the law is; where our views diverge is in our assessments of its future direction.

We appear to disagree on the purposes for which courts established the informed-consent doctrine as it now exists and on the extent to which current developments now affect the normal conduct of both research and prac-

---

[22]There are several examples in the last two years of mental health professionals and their associations taking the initiative in designing interdisciplinary mechanisms to protect patients' rights and well-being when the more extreme forms of treatment are proposed or the adequacy of consent is in doubt. Several professional associations submitted proposals for the revision of the *Wyatt v. Stickney* Standard (4, pp. 400-401), governing electroconvulsive therapy and aversive conditioning. In *Rogers v. Macht* (21) the Massachusetts Psychiatric Society submitted an *amicus* brief proposing the establishment of "treatment review boards," consisting of an attorney and two psychiatrists, to monitor the use of psychotropic medications in state hospitals. The Joint Task Force of the Florida Division of Retardation and the Florida State University Department of Psychology have proposed a model system for interdisciplinary and lay review of behavior therapy programs, published as a monograph (94). See also Halleck (95).

tice. In particular, however, we appear to differ on the very basic issue of the nature of intrafamilial relations and the degree to which courts have the power to and should enforce parental authority, if and when it may conflict with a child's autonomy. Until recently, courts at all levels were willing to protect the family as a unit from outside interference. In the absence of physical neglect or brutality, the legal system presumed almost conclusively that in parent-child relations involving decision making or potential psychological harm, the parent was right. In the last several years, some courts have begun to recognize that brutality to a child's spirit may be as devastating as physical brutality and to understand that this conflict does in fact arise in many households. The relevance of these decisions to the problems raised by proxy consent to research, however, is open to question.

The jurisprudential underpinnings of informed consent are theoretical concepts of self-determination and respect for autonomy which, if taken seriously by the courts issuing opinions on the subject, would indeed have revolutionized physician-patient and researcher-subject relationships and probably would affect all fiduciary relationships, including those between lawyer and client. However, such a promise or a threat, depending on one's viewpoint, has little actual likelihood of coming to pass.

There are two legal theories on which an action for informed consent could be based. If battery, defined as "unlawful touching," were invoked, treatment without consent would itself constitute the actionable wrong, regardless of the consequences. Thus, if a patient were not warned of the risks of a surgical procedure or of the side effects of a drug, had agreed to the treatment, and was restored to perfect health, the physician could still be found liable for violating the patient's right to autonomy. No physical damage need be proved in a battery case because the interest to be protected is a dignitary one. Almost unanimously, however, courts have refused to allow these claims to be heard in battery unless the patient gave no consent at all to the procedure (65, 96). In recent years, battery actions have in most, but not all, cases involved situations in which the wrong operation has been performed, usually after mix-ups in charts (97, 98).

Since negligence, "failure to use due care," has been accepted almost universally as the theory to be applied, an examination of the elements of any negligence action may indicate the limitations on the right to recover damages. It is quite clear under negligence law that no recovery of damages will be permitted, regardless of the magnitude of the lack of due care, unless the plaintiff-patient can prove that physical damage occurred (99, 100). There has never been a successful informed-consent case in which no physical harm had occurred. The same legal rule applies in other forms of malpractice actions and results in such rulings as a decision that a clearly negligent failure to diagnose a fracture is not compensable when the patient was put to bed and told to rest, if his condition was not aggravated by the delay (101, 102). To refer specifically to the example Dr. Stone uses, if the courts were seriously concerned with autonomy and self-determination, giving a patient a drug that could cause tardive dyskinesia without warning him of that possibility would, under battery law, give him a cause of action whether he developed the condition or not. Under negligence law, the patient would have to prove that he developed the condition and that it occurred more probably than not as the result of the drug (103, 104). Moreover, the patient usually would have to offer proof that a reasonably prudent patient with the same condition would have refused the treatment if he had known of this possibility (105, 106).

In addition, under the negligence standard, the only risks of therapy that must be disclosed are those classified as "material." Even in those states that adhere to the "prudent patient" standard of disclosure discussed by Dr. Stone and do not, therefore, require a patient to present expert medical testimony that a reasonably prudent physician in the community would have disclosed the particular risk, if there is any question that a risk is "material," expert testimony to that effect is required (109). Under battery law, where the thrust of the complaint is dignitary harm, materiality would be totally irrelevant.

Furthermore, although the doctrine of therapeutic privilege—the right of the physician to withhold information in the best medical interests of the patient—has been restricted by some decisions, it is and undoubtedly will remain a viable alternative to full disclosure in some cases. Interestingly enough, however, as Katz (108) has pointed out, insufficient reliable data exist about the consequences of disclosure on patients to arrive at the conclusion that it is likely to be generally harmful.

It would thus seem that the limitations imposed on the jurisprudential concepts of autonomy and self-determination theoretically expressed in the doctrine of informed consent, by virtue of its classification as a negligence action rather than as one in battery, have actually materially lessened the burdens of expectation imposed by law on the medical profession. If one views greater patient decision making as a threat to the physician-patient relationship, the actual holdings, compared with the rhetoric included as dicta in some of the opinions, indicate that this threat will not materialize.

The practical effects of informed-consent litigation to date appear to me to be negligible, aside from frightening physicians. It is, for example, quite clear in almost all cases in which awards to patients have been upheld on appeal that the treatment given was, if not legally negligent, at least clearly deficient, and the deficiency was also proved. Except for some product-liability actions against drug manufacturers decided under principles of strict liability, not under the principles applicable to a physician in a malpractice suit, I am aware of no cases dealing with a situation in which the patient was injured by a genuinely unpreventable, untoward occurrence. For example, in *Canterbury v. Spence* (109), supposedly a revolutionary departure from the previous law of informed consent, the patient was recovering normally from a laminectomy when he fell a day or two later. Paralysis followed the fall, not the surgery. In *Koury v. Follo* (64), one of the cases Dr. Stone cites on liability for drug reactions of which a patient is not warned, the defendant, a pediatrician, ordered the drug to be given in adult doses to a baby. Thus, while the patient's rights of self-determination and autonomy are a concern of the courts and should be the concern of thoughtful physicians, excessive fear of malpractice liability for failure to obtain adequately informed consent appears unjustified if one remembers that the extant cases have all occurred in situations where inadequate medical care was given. The reason, I believe, that there have been almost no "mal-research" cases is that medical researchers in university settings tend to be extremely competent physicians, and the careful follow-up care received by these patients prevents the same sort of carelessness from occurring.

In considering the application of the doctrine of informed consent, either actually or theoretically, to those persons for whom proxy consent must be given, the only groups for which this consent is required as a class are children and those adjudicated individually as legally incompetent. In all other categories, such as mental incompetence without a declaration of legal incompetence, the individual patient's capacity to consent is overriding. In minors, the personal capacity to understand is in many cases largely irrelevant. It thus appears that the general principles derived in determining the limits of proxy consent for infants and children can be applied in other contexts.

Dr. Stone questions the recent decisions restricting parental rights to commit children to mental institutions, to give consent for nontherapeutic research, and to veto a minor girl's consent to an abortion. I must respectfully dissent from his position that these decisions have interfered with legitimate family autonomy. In cases involving a minor girl's consent to an abortion or the institutional commitment of a child, the existing abuse of parental power in the home, as amply documented in many court decisions, would have had serious lifetime consequences for the child. I would totally remove these situations from the analogies Dr. Stone draws to such traditionally accepted responsibilities of parental decision making as bedtimes and household chores.

Parents are not always wise, decent, or understanding with their children, and the resulting psychological abuse may be far more brutal and harmful on a long-term basis than a physical beating, from which the law has always protected a child. For example, a parent who has vetoed his minor daughter's abortion has no legal duty whatever to support or care for her baby (110).

Should the baby be unadoptable for any reason, she, a minor, is the only person legally required to provide parental care for the child, although the baby's father is responsible for contributing to the baby's support. In the Massachusetts abortion case decided by the Supreme Court and criticized by Dr. Stone, the minor who wished to have the abortion had submitted uncontradicted testimony in the trial court to the effect that her father had told her that if she ever became pregnant he would kill the boy and throw her out of the house (111, 112) In a normal, loving household, parents do not commit their children to mental institutions for malicious reasons or in order to abandon them, but not all households are normal or loving, and the case law is replete with examples of situations where this has in fact occurred (113-117). The normal parent-child relationship is unlikely to be seriously affected by these decisions; the malicious or vicious parent may be.

There does not appear to be an analogous potential for abuse in the biomedical research environment, and thus the relevance of these decisions is questionable. The most liberal advocates of pediatric research would not normally argue in favor of using a child as a subject in any experiment in which the risk of harm (as is obviously present in an unnecessary, malicious commitment) substantially outweighs the expected benefits to the child himself.

Where the research is intended to benefit the particular child, there appears to be no question that the parent may consent to the same extent that the parent may consent to standard therapy. In fact, it is at least arguable, although there is no case law on the subject, that in a life-threatening situation where no standard therapy exists a parent would be guilty of neglect if he refused to allow a child to participate in available research that might alleviate the condition.

The proxy-consent issue in nontherapeutic research on children is normally framed in terms of whether a parent may consent to research in which the minor is exposed to "no discernible risk of harm" (118). The American Academy of Pediatrics, for example, has long advocated a more sensible system of drug testing on children than now exists, but its position paper excludes the possibility of Phase I testing on children (119). Although there are some ethicists and a few scientists who have felt, long before the recent Supreme Court decisions, that a parent may not consent to any nontherapeutic research on a child (120, 121), the American Medical Association's *Principles of Ethics*, most physicians, and some philosophers, notably, Richard McCormick, support the concept of proxy consent to research within the limitations of "no discernible risk of harm" (122). Until the *Nielsen* case (25) reaches a final determination, there will, however, be no case law directly on this subject. Since, as Dr. Stone points out, the family is left alone by the legal system to make its own decisions on bedtimes and boarding schools, it is most unlikely that courts would intervene to forbid a parent to consent to research on a child when it encompassed no greater risk of harm than those activities. The fact that the Supreme Court and lower courts have intervened to protect the child from such gross abuse as a denial of the right to abortion or a malicious commitment does not appear to indicate in the least that they would necessarily intervene where a parent has consented to the taking of a blood sample from his child.

However, a very specific and fairly unusual aspect of the *Nielsen* case (25) may make it a poor case on which to develop a legal principle. As Dr. Stone points out, in the protocol which is the subject of the suit, the parent of each child-subject would be paid approximately $300 to compensate him for transportation or other expenses incurred by the child's participation. This is unlikely to be considered simply "reimbursement" by a court because all the families would receive the same amount regardless of actual, documented expenses incurred. Such serious questions of both law and ethics are raised by any payment to a parent, as opposed to a savings bond or other compensation to the child, as to risk having a court invalidate such proxy consents (123, 124). These principles, however, do not apply to situations in which the consent is given without payment.

The legal system has for years been much more concerned with the child's financial protection vis-à-vis a parent or guardian than it has with the child's autonomy in relation to the same persons. For example, income from a trust of which a minor is a beneficiary may not be expended by a parent for his own use (125). Courts require strict accounting by guardians on an annual or semiannual basis of expenditures of a minor-ward's funds, whereas, unless there is evidence of actual abuse, the same courts never inquire into the environment the same guardian provides for the same child. Selling a child to adoptive parents is clearly illegal. Thus, although there is no litigation on this point to date, it is quite possible that a court might hold that payment to a parent, as opposed to payment to the child, might be sufficient to coerce a proxy consent, making such a consent invalid.

In sum, a qualitatively different issue, in which a court could reasonably find a conflict of interest, seems to be raised by cases in which payment is offered as contrasted with those in which it is not. The same principles would seem to apply to mentally incompetent adult patients for whom consent must be given by a guardian.

One fundamental principle of research ethics would seem to be that no incompetent (i.e., child, retarded person, or mentally ill person) should be used as a research subject if a competent adult is biologically qualified to be a subject in the research (126). For example, in the experiments on hepatitis vaccine among the children at Willowbrook (34), a great deal of the criticism centered around the fact that there was no reason that adults, such as the workers in the institution, could not have been appropriate subjects.

If the research, under the same conditions, had been in some way related to attempted alleviation of the children's handicaps, it is unlikely that it would have been criticized. Thus, where the research necessarily must be performed on the population of incompetents and is of substantial potential benefit to the subjects themselves, it would seem that, as long as no discernible harm can result, the validity of proxy consent is not open to serious legal question at this time. Where serious harm could result and where there is no potential benefit to the patient, I would hope that no incompetent would be selected, not from fear of the courts, but rather as a matter of ethics.

DR. STONE: Ms. Holder states that we "differ on the very basic issue of the nature of intrafamilial relations and the degree to which courts have the power to and should enforce parental authority, if and when it may conflict with a child's autonomy."

It is possible to cite cases like the Massachusetts abortion case and the *Willowbrook* case (34) which at face value are so repugnant that one cannot help but feel sympathy for the children involved, but I can easily cite countervailing facts which would arouse sympathy for parents. Ms. Holder does not claim to have engaged in an empirical study of the various fact situations, nor do I. Thus, argument at that level seems to me to be fruitless. I have argued that the court has no legal doctrine to guide it when it attempts to resolve intrafamilial disputes, that the child needs a continuing supportive environment in order to survive and grow, that the courts recognize that the family has a better chance of providing that environment than does the state. Therefore, they erect a presumption that assumes an identity of interests between parent and child because they are wary of entrenching on the family unit when there is no alternative. I hope Ms. Holder will deal with these questions to flesh out her disagreement with me about "the nature of intrafamilial relations and the degree to which courts have the power to and should enforce parental authority."

As to her argument that the extant cases of malpractice "have all occurred in situations where inadequate medical care was given," and that this explains the absence of malpractice research cases because research takes place in university settings where the quality of care is better, I simply disagree with her as to both assumptions. Anyone reading the Katz book (34) and the studies of research in prisons would know that a great deal of research has gone on outside of university settings, and was performed by physicians who were not "extremely competent." Further, although the consent issue is a way to get to the negligence problem, once the consent issue is established in law, it affects the standards of practice and has implications that, in my view, Ms. Holder simply minimizes or even ignores.

As to the rest of Ms. Holder's comments, I find it hard to believe that it is the $300 payment in the *Nielsen* case (25) that makes the difference, and if Professor Neilsen had really been concerned about it, I am sure that while he served on the Human Rights Committee he could have made the suggestion that the $300 be paid into a savings bond in the child's name. The money issue is simply a make-weight legal argument. The real issue is whether a parent can speak for his child as opposed to a court when no benefit is anticipated.

Mr. Scott suggests that "litigation has not brought psychopharmacologic research and treatment to a halt," and obviously that is correct in the sense that there are so few cases litigating research that it is impossible to contend that litigation per se has impeded research. However, one need only consider the fact that administrative agencies and legislatures are extremely sensitive to legal decisions. Indeed, often decisions become embodied in regulatory language. Recently, the federal prisons have cut back on all research, presumably on the theory that conditions in prisons are so coercive that prisoners cannot give informed consent. Similarly, lawyers working in departments of mental health all over the United States are interpreting the kind of decisions discussed by Mr. Scott in such a way that research becomes impossible. The adage that the law is a seamless web has many interpretations, and my argument is that the new regulations being produced everywhere reflect the thinking of the few decisions and the law review commentaries on those decisions.

Since Mr. Scott comments on the tone of my piece, I would like to comment on the tone of his. Essentially, his tone is that of Dr. Pangloss, and the presumption is that litigation has somehow led to orderly progress without significant costs. I think he is simply wrong about that. In the first place, there is a growing sentiment among lawyers of every stripe that federal courts have involved themselves in more than they can handle. Precedents set by mental health litigation are now being undermined by new decisions. Courts that eagerly embraced mental health litigation now seem eager to avoid it. The rate of turnover of professionals working in the public sector has accelerated so that there is almost no continuity of administration, treatment, or policy. Research in the public sector in neuropsychopharmacology is almost totally at an end, and constraints on new research projects are almost impossible to overcome. *Research and the Psychiatric Patient* (127) contains accounts by Jonathan Cole and others documenting the difficulty of neuropsychopharmacologic research based on regulation. It is in the context of this kind of regulation that I posed the question: What additional restraints should courts impose? Most of Mr. Scott's discussion is a reiteration of due process arguments, and he emphasizes the flexibility of due process standards. That, of course, is a well-known legal argument. However, flexible due process in theory becomes bureaucratic decision making in reality. I doubt very much that Mr. Scott would argue that the juvenile delinquent gets due process in law courts in the United States, and if his lawyer insists on it, either his present client will suffer, or the next ten clients he represents in that bureaucracy will suffer the judge's wrath. Counsel are restrained not only by the courts' limited time and crowded dockets, but by their traditional roles as I have described them.

Mr. Scott should be well aware of this since the Mental Health Law Project is now considering a case where the most elaborate due process safeguards imaginable were worked out by the higher courts and the current complaint is that lawyers representing mentally ill persons performed in a totally *pro forma* manner; thus, the disparity between the law in the books and the law in real life is so great as to make the arguments about due process almost meaningless.

As to Mr. Scott's contention that the lawyer will express the client's desires, that was not the question I was addressing. I have simply considered the question of what shall the lawyer do when his client is not competent to express his desires.

As to the many other roles in the mental health context that lawyers might fill, I am well aware of them, and have spelled them out in my monograph, Mental Health and Law: A System in Transition. Gov't Printing Office: Washington, D.C., 1975. I do not think that the Litwack article (87) and the Andalman and Chambers article (88) would convince anyone that there is considerable evidence that lawyers do play constructive roles in the mental health field, nor am I as sanguine as Mr. Scott that the bar will awaken to its responsibilities to the mentally disabled.

As to Mr. Scott's suggestions about what the neuropsychopharmacologic group could do, I think they are interesting and sensible. I wish he could have spelled out, however, how he would accommodate research objectives and the personal freedom of patients and subjects.

DR. GALLANT: As Dr. Stone has emphasized, the right to treatment has now become one of the major legal issues confronting psychiatric patient care in the courts. The concept of the right to treatment in an institution is derived from constitutional rights of liberty and should be specified as the individual's right to treatment or else to be released. Additionally, the patient has a constitutional right to be protected from "cruel and unusual punishments," thus from preventable deterioration in a private or state psychiatric institution. In the *Wyatt v. Stickney* case (4), it was argued that the court had the right to review the nature and duration of confinement of involuntarily committed persons. However, in establishing guidelines, it should be recognized by the courts that too much rigidity in the guidelines will hinder the experienced physician in his attempt to practice medicine in a manner that is superior to the accepted standard in his community.

An interesting opinion affecting the right to treatment was rendered by the Attorney General of the State of Louisiana (128). The opinion, which was a common-sense integration of the right of the patient to adequate treatment and the duty of the physician to use all available, efficacious treatment methods, stated:

> ... the duty to treat patients committed to a mental institution is expressly recognized by both state and federal courts. Those courts have held that patients who are committed to state mental hospitals have a constitutional right to receive such individual treatment that will give them a *realistic* opportunity to be cured or to improve. The purpose of Commitment is treatment, not merely custodial care ... The court in Welsh v. Likins, 373 F. Supp. 487, 1974 recently held that the constitutional right to receive proper treatment is a due process emanating from the Fourteenth Amendment of the U.S. Constitution.

The opinion thus approved, with the informed consent of the legally authorized representative, the use of "federally approved and regulated investigational drugs" in treating those schizophrenic patients who have not responded to standard available neuroleptic agents as part of the right to have "a realistic opportunity to be cured. . . "

The Constitution has now been interpreted by the courts as empowering the federal government with the judicial obligation to safeguard the constitutional rights of voluntarily confined persons in regard to due process. However, the question still remains whether or not the federal courts have the right to guarantee adequate medical treatment and the authority to propose specific guidelines and definitions on what constitutes adequate treatment. Practical problems did evolve from the *Wyatt* decision where the court issued thirty-five standards for the mental hospital and forty-nine for the state school, virtually covering hundreds of aspects of institutional care. Are the courts adequately staffed to permit comprehensive policing of these relatively large number of standards? As stated in Dr. Stone's response to the commentaries by Ms. Holder and Mr. Scott, the federal courts may have "involved themselves in more than they can handle." Another question arises about the judicial branch of government assuming executive functions which have traditionally been within the realm of the executive branch. In *Burnham v. Department of Public Health of Georgia* (129), the judge concluded that the patient did have a moral right to treatment, but the state did not have a legal obligation to provide treatment in the absence of a state statute. In this case, the federal court somehow decided that the Eleventh Amendment to the Constitution prohibited a federal order to require state expenditures.

Dr. Stone has also detailed the patient's right to refuse certain types of treatment. It is possible that in the near future even voluntary patients, including those who are mentally incompetent, will be allowed to refuse all forms of treatment that are not necessary to preserve life. In the case of *Bell v. Wayne County General Hospital at Eloise* (3), the federal court ruled that the involuntary patient confined under emergency procedures has the right to refuse surgery and electroconvulsive therapy (ECT) on nonreligious grounds, and may also refuse chemotherapy unless there is objective evidence that chemotherapy is clearly necessary to prevent physical injury to others.

At present, a regulation of the New York State Department of Mental Hygiene stipulates that voluntary patients may not be given treatment over their objections. In such a case, the patient must be discharged or, if appropriate, converted to involuntary status by court proceedings. In the case of minors, legal representation for the child is required at court hearings concerned with involuntary detention. There is no doubt that most psychiatrists, and probably most other physicians, do not wish to go through court procedures to convert the patient's status from voluntary to involuntary. This hesitation by psychiatrists could well result in the substitution of an inefficacious, benign treatment modality for an efficacious but somewhat perturbing treatment (e.g., ECT) or in premature release of their patients from the hospital, thus depriving them of adequate treatment. One study suggested that psychiatrists who feel threatened by legal challenges tend to decrease the quality of their clinical care of patients (130). When psychiatric commitment was challenged by lawyers on behalf of their patient-clients in a New York City public hospital, the physicians showed a marked trend to discharge the patients to avoid court appearances. These premature discharges occurred despite the fact that the judges in these cases universally tended to support psychiatric decisions and despite the fact that the discharged patients were at least as sick as patients whose commitments were unchallenged and had remained hospitalized. It is quite obvious that psychiatrists must be more adequately trained in the legal aspects of commitment and related procedures and that a more comfortable relationship between the legal respresentative of the patient and the mental health professional has to be developed.

Another point of view in regard to the right to treatment has been expressed by Chodoff (131). Chodoff discusses the right of the patient to be protected as well as to be treated. He offers an example of a severely depressed female patient who refuses to eat or refuses treatment because, "I don't deserve it." He questions whether or not her fellow man should allow her to die of starvation or share some responsibility for her treatment until her mental condition is adequate to make a competent and informed decision about her future. Even the libertarian lawyers would agree that this individual should have involuntary treatment to preserve her life and that an ongoing evaluation of her mental capacity to evaluate treatment should be part of the treatment process. Past court decisions have allowed doctors to override the expressed wishes of their patients where the treatment they sought to impose was intended to protect not the patient, but a third party or the public in general (132, 133,). Is it theoretically possible to use these precedents for ordering compulsory treatment for those individuals who may have severe suicidal or for that matter homicidal tendencies? There is no doubt that the individual, as in the cases cited, would then be denied due process as stated in the Fourteenth Amendment. However, uniform and consistent application of the Fourteenth Amendment in an attempt to protect the patient from deprivation of liberty or from harmful therapy can result in protecting the same patient from receiving adequate treatment. The availability of an advisory board composed of a patient legal surrogate, a family member if available, and an outside expert in psychiatry would be one solution for this very common problem. It is Chodoff's opinion that if we were to follow literally the advice of Szasz—"we shall value liberty more highly than mental health no matter how defined"—we would merely be absolving ourselves of moral responsibility for our fellow man (131). Chodoff discusses the right of the mentally ill to be protected from others as well as his right to treatment. He gives the example of a depressed senile person who might be permitted to conduct his financial affairs with an individual of questionable honesty. Again, an available protection committee for the patient would be able to evaluate this situation in a more adequate manner than the patient and possibly be more objective than the treating psychiatrist.

It should be recognized by laymen as well as by professionals that mental illness is not a myth or peculiar only to our society. Detailed and extensive work by Murphy concerning the incidence of schizophrenia in Eskimo tribes and in the Yorubans confirms the opinion that mental illness, particularly schizophrenia, is a worldwide disease with approximately the same incidence in all cultures (134). To absolve ourselves of responsibility for the mentally ill by claiming that the illness is a myth or to discharge them from the hospital prematurely to avoid judicial procedures might be comparable to turning aside a senile patient with severe memory loss who is incapable of caring for himself.

There is no doubt that "mental illness" is frequently misdiagnosed and commitment procedures can be subject to abuse. These deficiencies emphasize the need for training professional "patient surrogates" in the fields of law and psychiatry to serve as permanent members of what may be called Professional Review Committees or Treatment Review Committees. The development of third-party representation between the patient and the treatment staff of the institution is now becoming a reality.

Along with the trend in the direction of patient protection, a tendency has developed to lump various modalities of therapy together such as psychosurgery, psychopharmacologic agents, and ECT with the introduction of such terms as "chemical or physical straightjackets" which ignore the scientific evidence of the therapeutic efficacy for both drugs and ECT in the treatment of schizophrenia and depression (135). Extensive and well-controlled studies of the use of drug therapy and ECT in schizophrenia leave no doubt as to the significantly superior efficacy of these two treatment modalities compared to psychotherapy with schizophrenics. The emotional reactions against ECT by some lawyers involved in protecting the rights of patients hospitalized in institutions and the resultant legislation to restrict ECT (131) have not only been shocking, but detrimental to the treatment of the very patients they are trying to protect. As a result, these patients are now protected from receiving adequate treatment. As detailed in the study by Kumasaka et al. (130), most psychiatrists tend to avoid legal procedures, even if this results in inadequate treatment for the patient. Perhaps, some physicians, including psychiatrists, are to be blamed for the development of some of these problems which prevent patients from receiving adequate treatment. As Dr. Stone (136) has pointed out, the right-to-treatment decisions were at first ignored by psychiatrists and leading experts such as Katz who wrote an article in 1969 entitled "The right to treatment: An enchanting legal fiction" (137). The defensiveness of the psychiatrists only serves to prod the legal profession into overreactions to the profession of psychiatry.

Dr. Stone has proffered one possible solution to protect the patient from institutionalization without adequate treatment: to limit commitment to those hospitals approved by the Joint Commission on Accreditation of Hospitals which requires standards quite similar to those decreed in the *Wyatt* case (136). However, this type of private corporation may be subject to too many external pressure groups and would only serve to complicate the federal compliance procedures state and private mental hospitals will have to meet in order to be eligible for future National Health Insurance. An alternative would be the collaboration of the federal government with the state governments to initiate their own Joint Commission for Accreditation, consisting of state and federal representatives and utilizing a peer-review system in the same manner as is currently done for the review of federal training and research grant applications. If some proper solution is not found to decrease the recent trend toward intensifying the conflict between the treatment institutions and the committed patients, the final result may be that many patients may receive inadequate treatment as a result of premature discharge from hospitals. I do believe that Dr. Stone's statements about the eventual solution are valid: " . . . in the end the real solution to the problems addressed by the right to treatment cannot come from complicated judicial discourse about civil rights and civil liberties. It must come in a form of a system of national health insurance that includes adequate mental health coverage for inpatient as well as outpatient treatment and for chronic as well as acute mental illness. To some, this will seem unrealistic or too expensive or too much like socialized medicine. But is there a humane alternative that psychiatrists can endorse?" (136).

Dr. Stone has referred to Judge Johnson's prohibition of the use of proxy consent without legal precedent. Before proceeding further, we should consider an acceptable definition of informed consent, which is the prerequisite to competent research and treatment. There are three basic elements of informed consent: (a) legal capacity to give consent; (b) voluntary consent; and (c) sufficient knowledge of the nature of the procedure, its risks, and alternative treatments, if any (138). A number of courts have already insisted that consent forms include a disclosure of the existence and characteristics of alternative therapies (109).

Even with sincere attempts to obtain informed consent from adults, the results may be unsatisfactory for both the patient and the physician and/or investigator. Two studies of informed consent in voluntary patients admitted to the hospital indicated that the majority of them did not have an adequate understanding of the voluntary admission form they had signed (139, 140). While such studies reveal how difficult it is to fully inform a patient, they indicate as well that all mental hospital personnel should give voluntary patients individual notice of their status and rights at frequent intervals and such notices should be posted on all wards. Further, these studies underscore the need for professional full-time patient surrogates, who should be available to evaluate the patient's understanding of his legal rights. In this manner, the problem of informed consent can be addressed rather than dismissed by inferring that it is an impossible goal to attain.

Concerning confidentiality of patient research and treatment records, more recent court decisions and federal regulations have served to give additional protection to the patient and the researcher. In California, it has been ruled that an academic researcher has the same right to protect confidential sources of information as does the journalist (141). In the Federal Register of July 1, 1976, confidentiality of alcohol and drug-abuse patient records was considered to be a legal requirement except as defined in the exclusions cited in the regulation. No records of identity, diagnosis, prognosis, or treatment mentioned in connection with any drug-abuse prevention may be used to initiate or substantiate any criminal charges against the patient or to conduct any investigation of the patient (142). Labeling patients with diagnoses has resulted in an abridgement of the legal rights of psychiatric patients, particularly in regard to revealing the confidentiality of the psychiatric diagnoses and labels. In one review of the problem, Ennis (143) pointed out that the label or designation of "ex-mental patient" could result in the denial of housing in a public development without a special dispensation. In fact, in

Long Beach, Long Island, the patient was not even permitted to register in a public hotel.

There is no doubt that recent Federal District Court rulings such as in *Wyatt v. Stickney* (4) in Alabama have helped to improve the care of institutionalized patients. However, in this same case, which has accomplished much good, we also see how the intelligent physician is hindered when we come to the court guidelines which utilize the Physician's Desk Reference (PDR) for maximal dosages. Since it is well recognized in clinical pharmacology that individual patients may require considerably different dosages of medication due to genetic-metabolic differences in absorption, metabolism, and excretion, the use of the PDR dosage guidelines can be quite inappropriate and harmful to a considerable number of patients. In setting guidelines to decrease the mistakes of the incompetent physician, the court unfortunately also prevented the knowledgeable physician from using his expertise for the patient's welfare.

Another unfortunate hinderance to patient care developed as a result of the guidelines in the *Wyatt* case. Reimbursement for work was one of the requirements of the court decrees and patients were no longer able to participate in work therapy since institutions did not have necessary funds for work compensation. Subsequently, this oversight was corrected by the court's permitting patients to perform uncompensated labor for therapeutic purposes. Obviously, continuing judicial supervision is required in such instances as the *Wyatt* decision. As one of the psychopharmacologic consultants to the Partlow Human Rights Committee in the *Wyatt* case, I had the opportunity to observe the value of continuing court supervision. A notification of our forthcoming visit to inspect the charts at Partlow was associated with the elimination of the use of neuroleptic agents in approximately 400 patients within a two-month interval from the time of notification of our visit to the time of our inspection. Thus, the mere existence of an ongoing Human Rights Committee, representing continuing court supervision, serves to instill caution in the institutional personnel.

Our society does not offer recognition or increased status to the person who participates in medical research. Thus, if medical research is to continue and progress, our society will have to revise its present values extensively so that such participation will be respected and encouraged. Until that time, temporary efforts such as governmental responsibility for the financial liability of competent researchers, governmental financial support for training of patient surrogates and consultation by professional experts, and increased independence of Human Research Committees are absolute necessities if medical research is to survive.

Steps toward accomplishing some of these suggestions were recently recommended by the American Bar Association's (ABA) House of Delegates during the 1976 annual meeting (144). The House of Delegates recommended "absolute immunity" from civil liability to all members of medical disciplinary boards as well as to the witnesses, full confidentiality of such proceedings, and voluntary use of arbitration panels with the full knowledge that the panel's decision would be final and binding. Similar support of the Institutional Review Boards (IRBs) would contribute toward increasing the independence of these boards, a point strongly emphasized by Mr. Scott in his commentary. Deferred proposals of the ABA dealt with such subjects as setting of lawyers' contingency fees by court order and decreasing percentages of contingency fee schedules. Adoption of these recommendations by the federal and state governments would partially help to solve the recent malpractice litigation dilemma while still protecting the patient. Extension of similar governmental responsibility for liability for competent Human Research Committees and individual investigators is also required to allow research to progress while simultaneously protecting the subject. In this way, the increase of independence of the IRBs or Human Research Committees would contribute toward an acceptable accommodation between the researcher and the patient surrogate.

Although Dr. Stone is correct when he states that a great deal of research occurs outside of university settings, Ms. Holder's reasons for the lack of "mal-research" cases in university settings appear to have some validity. She stated that "medical researchers in university settings tend to be extremely competent physicians, and the careful follow-up care received by these patients prevents . . . carelessness from occurring." A recent summary of research risks in the sciences apparently confirms this opinion (145). The study showed that the injury rates among subjects in nontherapeutic research programs were lower than accidental injury rates among the general population and that the injury rates in therapeutic research were lower than the injury and fatality rates in nonexperimental treatments given in the hospitals. Thus, few lawsuits have resulted from clinical psychopharmacologic research, particularly within research institutes and university settings. However, recent regulatory restrictions in the Federal Register and DHEW guidelines have set additional limits on the researcher-subject relationship. Thus, the research investigator should be more concerned with the regulatory issues than with recent court decisions or litigation-minded patients. In those research projects by competent investigators that have been approved by appropriate IRBs (or Human Research Committees) and judged by these boards to have potential valuable benefits for the patient as well as society, future legislation will have to protect the researchers as well as the patients by enabling the investigators to accomplish their work without fear of inappropriate litigation. The present judicial trend toward requiring independent medical expert consultation, making legal counsel available for patient and staff consultation, and providing legal guardians for certain types of patients with limited mental capacity imposes an impossible financial burden on the researcher. Therefore, if competent research is to continue, then financial support for such patient protection will have to be made available by federal and state sources. It is in these areas that the research psychopharmacologist should become more knowledgeable and more concerned.

DR. LEVINE: I should like to comment on the patient surrogate/patient advocate issue. At least four times in the above discussion we have been told that patient surrogates, advocates, or ombudsmen are inevitable. I don't see the inevitability, and I don't see the general utility or necessity for such people. In the research context, we see these people are being recommended to supervise the negotiations for informed consent. In proposed DHEW regulations, for example, Consent Committees are assigned this function for all subjects in various broad categories—e.g., the institutionalized mentally infirm. In general, the presence of such persons would tend to undermine the purposes of informed consent and the reasons it was set up in the first place.

I don't agree with Dr. Stone's analysis of why we have informed consent. I think it is supposed to have to do with respecting the person's ability and prerogative to make an independent decision as to how to dispose of himself or herself. If you say to this person, "You must have a third party here, a third party whom we have selected and employed to look over your decision," this is tantamount to saying that we suspect that you may be irresponsible, incompetent, unable to comprehend, or irrational. This seems to be incompatible with the legal or ethical theories underlying the requirement for informed consent.

I do recognize that there is a need for such people in some situations. However, except in very unusual circumstances, the subject should have the right to select the third party. Does that person want a doctor for a medical opinion, a lawyer for a legal opinion, or an uncle for advice of a family sort? The prospective subject or patient should be allowed to select that person; and only in very extraordinary circumstances would I require a third party to look into the situation.

I would not attempt to identify these classes of activities in regulations. Rather, I would assign responsibility to the IRB to decide on a protocol-by-protocol basis the need for a third party, who should select the third party, and whether the third party should be mandatory or optional.

DR. WYATT: As a clinician researcher, I am very pleased that so many serious and thoughtful people are attempting to use formal techniques for answering the questions that must be answered every day on our wards. For most of us, these decisions are made without the benefit of detailed study of academic philosophy or legal precedent. The advantage of having others discuss these issues is that the burden of making many complicated decisions is placed on a much broader base than it has been in the past. Thus, the responsiblity is shared, although not in a legal sense, but a human one. From my point of view, researchers will gain as much or more benefit from this as our patients. It is of some interest to me, however, that the patients and their families are rarely asked to represent themselves in these discussions. It is, after all, the patient and his family who have the most to lose from a researcher's indiscretions as well as the most to gain from any progress in prevention or treatment.

So many issues have been touched upon that responding to them all would take every bit as much consideration as the authors put into their own deliberations. One issue in particular, however, caught my eye.

The patient advocate trained in combined medical-legal programs seems to be an important concept. My immediate response is that all patients can use as much help as we can give them in making crucial life decisions. For example, it would help me if I had an advocate trained in mechanical-legal issues to negotiate the price of repairs on my ten-year-old car with my mechanic. With somewhat more thought, however, I begin to wonder just what the medically-legally trained patient advocate might accomplish.

Before I give a patient a drug, I now go through the following procedures: I decide whether the project is worthy of my time as well as the risk-benefit to the patient; ask my collaborator's opinion; submit the protocol to the appropriate hospital review board, the drug company supplying the drug, the Food and Drug Administration, a granting agency, the patient's doctor, his family, and, from time to time, a public defender. When the project is completed, its merits are reviewed by journal referees, editors, and professional colleagues. In my experience, everybody on this list wants to protect the patient's rights. Thus, while I think that the patient advocate might prove useful, before recommending large-scale training and use of such people, I would like to see better defined what the advocate will be doing that is not already being done. Also, who would have an advocate and what part would the patient play in choosing his own, or for that matter, whether he has one? Finally, let's determine their benefit on a small scale using the rigorous procedures that we apply to our own science.

DR. GALLANT: I would like to add just one comment which I was going to suggest later in Dr. Lebacqz's chapter. If the IRBs or Human Research Committees did have the right to decide on a protocol-by-protocol basis when a patient surrogate was necessary, such as with severely ill, schizophrenic patients, perhaps the decision-making process of the reviewing committees would be improved if the IRBs were obligated to report their proceedings on such cases to a central clearinghouse. The periodic reporting of the proceedings and decisions would serve to educate the boards and the public about how the various committees develop their decision-making policies in particular cases. Such a periodic summary report would help to develop uniformity of procedures, ethical guidelines, and decisions. There is no reason why these IRBs, most of which receive their funding either directly or indirectly via government grants, should not immediately be assigned the obligation to report to this type of central clearinghouse.

MR. FORCE: I want to make one thing perfectly clear. I think all of us ought to bear in mind the limitations of the law. It is very easy to pass a statute or adopt a regulation. Whether or not that statute or regulation will have the intended impact is really quite something else, and I find myself being somewhat sympathetic to Dr. Levine's remarks. He said that even if you had patient advocates, surrogates, etc., who are they? What would they do? What can we expect to come from them?

As a result of the Miranda case (146), law enforcement officers are required to advise arrestees of their right to remain silent and their right to an attorney, etc., in order to prevent a coercive atmosphere for interrogation; but we have found that empirically it just doesn't have that impact.

I am not suggesting that the various legal proposals made here will not necessarily work, but I think that we ought to have at least a healthy skepticism in that regard. There are many areas where we have been unable to protect individual rights despite extensive litigation and judicial activism. In regard to the rights of suspected criminals, not only has there been a lack of impact from the Miranda decision, but also we have been unable to protect individual privacy by judicial implementation of the Fourth Amendment (147, 148). Prison reform litigation is another example where courts have been of limited utility in safeguarding human rights (149). Therefore, it is probably a mistake to assign too much responsibility to litigation as a means for protecting the rights of research subjects and patients.

This is not to say that courts have no role to play. The question is not whether courts should play a role in defining the limits of research and treatment, but what role they should play. That question should be answered only after considering the realities implicit in the limitations of judicial action. In evaluating the success of judicial action, the relevant concern is not how many research projects or treatment modalities have been prohibited or prematurely terminated, but rather to what extent litigation has advanced the human dignity of the actual or potential subjects and patients.

Legal institutions can only be effective through the formulation and application of standards directed to specified objectives. While I basically agree with Dr. Stone's positions, I believe that it is unnecessary to posit the "due process" standard in opposition to the "cruel and unusual punishment" standard.

Traditionally, due process may be invoked to protect rights in several different ways. Most often, due process may ensure that a person will not be adversely affected unless the decision to affect his personal interests has been arrived at fairly (150-152). This aspect of due process focuses on the procedures that surround the decision-making process. Certainly no one would quarrel with the assertion that the process for deciding to use particular subjects in psychopharmacologic research should be a fair one. But what does "fairness" mean in this context? It need not imply all the ritual that accompanies a criminal trial. It need not necessarily involve an adversary process (153). In routine situations, it is suggested that due process is satisfied when a research protocol has been approved by a peer group such as an IRB and the selection of subjects is either with their consent or is not arbitrary and unreasonable if they are unable to consent, i.e., the process may not be characterized by overreaching. In the case of children, it is suggested that with the absence of circumstances indicating a conflict of interest or reasonably suggesting inquiry as to the likelihood of conflict of interest parental consent is neither arbitrary nor unreasonable and should be considered as satisfying due process.

Due process requirements, in the procedural sense, should be explicit. The researcher, the attorney, and the judge must be able to distinguish between permissible and impermissible procedures with relative ease in most cases. Vague references to "privacy" or to the First Amendment are insufficient, and the case-by-case approach creates too much uncertainty for the researcher.

Procedural considerations should be separated from a second form of due process that might also constrain research or treatment. If we assume that a research subject, although of doubtful competence, has consented to participate in a research project that has therapeutic implications for his condition and, further, that his family and legal guardian have consented, and if his attorney can show no violation of required legal procedures, then are there still circumstances where a court might find that the research project would violate the subject's rights? I think so. The *Kaimowitz* case (5) comes close to this situation. Notwithstanding full compliance with the procedural requirements of due process, there are situations in which research or treatment should and would be prohibited under due process because it creates an unreasonable invasion of the subject's human dignity.

I don't think that we can create legal standards in this area by abstractly pointing to the rights of privacy or freedom of thought. In evaluating the subject's dignity in these situations, judges and lawyers are on thin ice because balancing benefits and risks and weighing societal interests calls for sensitive and complex decision making. For a court to make these decisions, it is necessary to evaluate scientific as well as humane considerations and to measure these against the appropriate legal standard. To use "privacy" or the "right to be let alone" as the legal standard begs the question. The legal standard, since it must be applied to "scientific facts" that are never completely comprehensible to the courts, should exclude research or treatment only where the interests of society in preserving the dignity or privacy of the individual clearly outweigh any problematical gain to him or to society. Here, the suggestion that we draw an analogy to the "cruel and unusual punishment" standard used in criminal law would appear to be sound (154).

Under this approach, the court would seek to determine, (a) based on existing knowledge, (b) viewing the situation through the eyes of a person of reasonable sensitivity, (c) with due regard for the subject or patient, whether the research or treatment "shocks the conscience"—that is, does the research or treatment expose the subject or patient to risk, pain, or discomfort that is excessive, considering readily available alternatives and prospective benefits to the individual and to society at large? Admittedly, this standard is far from precise, but it at least would circumscribe research or treatment that could be characterized as "outrageous."

REFERENCES

1. *Wyatt v. Aderholt,* 368 F. Supp. 1382 (M.D. Ala. 1973), Supp. order, 368 F. Supp. 1383 (J.D. Ala. 1974).
2. *Wade v. Bethesda Hospital,* 356 F. Supp. 380 (S.D. Ohio 1973).
3. *Bell v. Wayne County General Hospital at Eloise,* 384 F. Supp. 1085 (E.D. Mich. 1974).
4. *Wyatt v. Stickney,* 344 F. Supp. 387 (M.D. Ala. 1972), *aff'd in part* sub nom. *Wyatt v. Aderholt,* 503 F. 2d 1905 (5th Cir. 1974).
5. *Kaimowitz v. Department of Mental Health of the State of Michigan,* Civ. No. 73-19434 AW (Cir. Ct., Wayne County, Mich., July 10, 1973). (All references are to slip opinion.) This decision was not published officially but may be found in two casebooks: Miller, W., Dawson, R.O., Dix, G.E., and Parnas, R.I. *The Mental Health Process,* 2nd ed. Mineola, N.Y.: New York Foundation Press, 1976, p. 567. And Brooks, A.D. *Law, Psychiatry and the Mental Health System.* Boston: Little, Brown, 1974, p. 902.
6. *Mackey v. Procunier,* 477 F. 2d 877 (9th Cir. 1973).
7. *Weidenfeller v. Kidulis,* 380 F.S. 445 (E.D. Wis. 1974).
8. Wexler, D. Token and taboo: Behavior modification, token economics, and the law. *Cal. Law Rev.,* 61:81, 1973.
9. Cole, J.O., and Davis, J.M. Clinical efficacy of the phenothiazines as antipsychotic drugs. In: *Psychopharmacology: A Review of Progress 1957-1967.* Daniel H. Efron, ed. Washington, D.C.: Public Health Service Publication, 1968, pp. 1057-1063.
10. Lehmann, H.E. Problems in controlled clinical evaluations, in *Psychopharmacology: A Review of Progress 1957-1967.* Daniel H. Efron, ed. Washington, D.C.: Public Health Service Publication, 1968, p. 952.

11. Gross, M. et al. Discontinuation of treatment with ataractic drugs. In: *Recent Advances in Biological Psychiatry.* J. Wortis, ed. New York: Grune & Strattone, 1961, pp. 3, 44.

12. National Institute of Mental Health–Psychopharmacology Service Center Collaborative Study Group. Phenothiazine treatment in acute schizophrenia: Effectiveness. *Arch. Gen. Psychiat.,* 10:246, 1964.

13. *Lessard v. Schmidt,* 349 F. Supp. 1073 (E.D. Wisc. 1972). Judgment vacated and case remanded for further consideration in light of *Huffman v. Pursue, Ltd.,* 420 U.S. 592 (1975).

14. Katz, J., Goldstein, J., and Dershowitz, A. *Psychoanalysis, Psychiatry, and Law.* New York: The Free Press, 1967, pp. 423-459.

15. Brief of *Amicus Curiae,* American Orthopsychiatric Association et al., for the reconsideration of the Court's order of February 28, 1975, *Wyatt v. Hardin,* CA No. 3195-N.

16. *Wyatt v. Hardin,* CA No. 3195-N, Supp. order (D.C. M.D. Ala. 1975).

17. Caldwell, A., and Brodie, S. Enforcement of the Criminal civil rights statute, 18 U.S.C. 242, in prison brutality cases. *Geo. Law J.,* 52:706, 1964.

18. Jacob, B. Prison discipline and inamtes' rights. *Harvard Civ. Rights-Civ. Lib. Law Rev.,* 5:227, 1970.

19. *Jobson v. Henne,* 355 F. 2d 129 (2 Civ. 1966).

20. *Donaldson v. O'Connor,* 422 U.S. 563 (1975).

21. *Rogers v. Macht,* CA 75-161OT, hearing slated on preliminary injunction motion (D.C. Mass.).

22. *Nelson v. Heyne,* 491 F. 2d 352 (7th Cir. 1974).

23. *NYARC v. Rockefeller,* 357 F. Supp. 752 (E.D. N.Y. 1973).

24. *Winters v. Miller,* 446 F. 2d 65 (2nd Cir.), cert. denied 404 U.S. 985 (1971).

25. *Nielsen v. The Regents of the University of California,* Civ. No. 665-049 (S.F. Super. Ct. filed Sept. 11, 1973).

26. Konkle, B. *Nielsen v. The Regents:* Children as pawns or persons. *Hastings Const. Law Quart.,* 2:1151-1176, Fall, 1975.

27. *Bartley v. Kremens,* 402 F. Supp. 1039 (U.S.D.C., E. Pa.), *probable juris. noted* 44 LW 2063.

28. *Meyer v. Nebraska,* 262 U.S. 390 (1923).

29. *Pierce v. Society of Sisters,* 268 U.S. 510, 534-535 (1925).

30. *Stanley v. Illinois,* 405 U.S. 645, 651 (1972).

31. *Skinner v. Oklahoma,* 316 U.S. 535, 541 (1942).

32. *May v. Andersun,* 345 U.S. 528, 533 (1953).

33. *Wisconsin v. Yoder,* 406 U.S. 205, 232 (1972).

34. Katz, J. *Experimentation with Human Beings.* New York: Russell Sage Foundation, 1972.

35. *Planned Parenthood of Central Missouri v. Danforth,* 44 USLW 5197 at 5204 (1976).

36. *Mackey v. Procunier,* 477 F. 2d 877, 878 (9th Cir. 1973).

37. *Knecht v. Gillman,* 488 F. 2d 1136 (8th Cir. 1973).

38. Shapiro, M. Legislating the control of behavior control: Autonomy and coercive use of organic therapies. *So. Cal. Law Rev.,* 47:237, 1974.

39. *Roe v. Wade,* 410 U.S. 113 (1973).

40. Utah Code Ann. Sec. 76-7-305 (Interim Supp. 1975).

41. Cal. Welf. and Institutions Code Sec. 5325 (f)-(g) (West Supp. 1976).
42. Ingelfinger, F.J. Informed (but uneducated) consent. *New Eng. J. Med.*, 287: 465, 1972.
43. Barber, B., Lally, J.J., Makarushka, J.L., and Sullivan, D. *Research on Human Subjects.* New York: Russell Sage Foundation, 1973.
44. Gray, B.H. *Human Subjects in Medical Experimentation.* New York: John Wiley & Sons, 1975.
45. Glass, E.S. Restructuring informed consent: Legal therapy for the doctor-patient relationship. *Yale Law J.*, 79:1533, 1969-70.
46. Prosser, W. *Torts*, pp. 34-37, 102-107, 161-166, and Chap. 2, Sec. 9, 4th ed., 1971.
47. Restmt. (2d) *Torts*, Sec. 13 (1965).
48. *Mohr v. Williams*, 95 Minn. 261, 104 N.W. 12 (1904).
49. Fried, C.: *Medical Experimentation: Personal Integrity and Social Policy.* Amer. Elsevier Publishing Co., New York, 1974, p. 23.
50. *Hart v. Brown*, 289 A. 2d 386 (Conn. 1972).
51. *Masden v. Harrison*, No. 6865 (Eq. Mass. Sup. Jud. Ct., June 12, 1957).
52. *Foster v. Harrison*, No. 6874 (Eq. Mass. Sup. Jud. Ct., Nov. 20, 1957).
53. *In re Richardson*, No. 6091 (La. Cir. Ct. App., Oct. 22, 1973).
54. Skegg, P. Consent to medical procedures on minors. *Modern Law Rev.*, 36:370, 1973.
55. *Strunk v. Strunk*, 445 S.W. 2d, 145 (Ky. 1969).
56. American College of Neuropsychopharmacology. *Statement of Principles of Ethical Conduct for Neuropsychopharmacologic Research in Human Subjects.* June, 1976. Reprinted in *this volume*, Chapter I.
57. *Cooper v. Roberts*, 220 Pa. Super. 260, 267, 286 A. 2d 647, 650 (1971), Pa. Stat. Ann. tit. 40, Secs. 1301.101-.1006 (Supp. 1976).
58. *Scaria v. St. Paul Fire and Marine Insurance Company*, 68 Wis. 2d 1, 227 N.W. 2d 647 (1975).
59. *Wilkinson v. Vesey*, 110 R.I. 606, 295 A. 2d 676 (1972).
60. *Canterbury v. Spence*, 464 F. 2d 772 (D.C. Cir.), cert. denied, 409 U.S. 1064 (1972).
61. *Natanson v. Kline*, 187 Kan. 186, 354 P. 2d 670 (1960).
62. *Incollingo v. Ewing*, 444 Pa. 263, 274-275, 282 A. 2d 206, 213 (1971).
63. *Sharpe v. Pugh*, 155 S.E. 2d 108 (N.C. 1967).
64. *Koury v. Follo*, 158 S.E. 2d 548 (N.C. 1968).
65. *Trogun v. Fruchtman*, 209 N.W. 2d 297 (Wis. 1973).
66. *Wyatt v. Stickney*, 325 F. Supp. 781 (M.D. Ala. 1971). 334 F. Supp. 1341 (M.D. Ala. 1971), 344 F. Supp. 373 and 387 (M.D. Ala. 1972), *aff'd. in part, modified in part sub nom. Wyatt v. Aderholt*, 503 F. 2d 1305 (5th Cir. 1974).
67. *Scott v. Plante*, 532 F. 2d 939 (3d Cir. 1976).
68. *Price v. Sheppard*, 239 N.W. 2d 905 (Minn. 1976).
69. *Wyatt v. Hardin*, Civ. No. 3195-N (M.D. Ala., Order dated Feb. 28, 1975, modified July 1, 1975) *(semble)*, reproduced in *Mental Disability Law Rep.*, 1:55, 1976.
70. *Stanley v. Georgia*, 394 U.S. 557, 565-566 (1969).
71. *Whitree v. State*, 56 Misc. 2d 693, 699, 290 N.Y.S. 2d 486, 501 (Ct. Cl. 1968).
72. *Nason v. Superintendent of Bridgewater State Hospital*, 393 Mass. 313, 233 N.E. 2d 908, 910 (1968).
73. *Roe v. Wade*, 410 U.S. 113, 154 (1973).

74. *Brady v. United States,* 397 U.S. 742, 756 (1970).
75. *Johnson v. Zerbst,* 304 U.S. 458, 464 (1938).
76. *Wisconsin v. Yoder,* 406 U.S. 205, 214-215, 221-229 (1972).
77. *Sherbert v. Verner,* 374 U.S. 398, 403, 406-409 (1963).
78. *Cleveland Board of Education v. LaFleur,* 414 U.S. 632 (1974).
79. *Shelton v. Tucker,* 364 U.S. 479 (1960).
80. Friedman, P. Legal regulation of applied behavioral analysis in mental institutions and prisons. *Ariz. Law Rev.,* 17:39, 72-74, 1975.
81. *Donaldson v. O'Connor,* 422 U.S. 563, 575 (1975), citing *Shelton v. Tucker* (79).
82. *Wolff v. McDonnell,* 418 U.S. 539 (1974).
83. *Goldberg v. Kelley,* 397 U.S. 254 (1970).
84. *Goss v. Lopez,* 419 U.S. 565, 581 (1975).
85. *In re Gault,* 387 U.S. 1 (1967).
86. *Doe v. Younger,* Civ. No. 14407 (Calif., 4th App. Dist., Apr. 23, 1976).
87. Litwack, T. The role of counsel in civil commitment proceedings: Emerging problems. *Cal. Law Rev.,* 62:816, 823-827, 1974.
88. Andalman, L., and Chambers, D. Effective counsel for persons facing civil commitment: A survey, a polemic and a proposal. *Miss. Law J.,* 45:43, 62-69, 1974.
89. Brief of Department of the Public Advocate, Division of Mental Health Advocacy, State of New Jersey as *Americus Curiae* in *Kremens v. Bartley,* probable jurisdiction noted, U.S., 96 S. Ct. 1456 (1976).
90. *State ex rel. Memmel v. Mundy,* Civ. No. 441-417 (Cir. Ct., Milwaukee County, Aug. 18, 1976).
91. Sprague, R., and Werry, J. Methodology of psychopharmacological studies with the retarded. *Int. Rev. Res. Mental Retard.,* 5:147, 1971.
92. Marker, G. Phenothiazines and the mentally retarded: Institutional drug abuse? MHLP Summary of Activities. March, 1975.
93. Marholin, D. and Philips, D. Methodological issues in psychopharmacological research: Chlorpromazine—a case in point. *Amer. J. Orthopsychiat.,* 46:477, 1976.
94. Joint Task Force of the Florida Division of Retardation and Florida State University Department of Psychology. *M.R. Research—Guidelines for the Use of Behavioral Procedures in State Programs for Retarded Persons.* National Association for Retarded Citizens, 1975.
95. Halleck, S. Legal and ethical aspects of behavior control. *Am. J. Psychiat.,* 131: 381, 1974.
96. *Dow v. Kaiser Foundation Hospitals, Cal. Rptr.* 90:747 (Cal. 1970).
97. *Bryson v. Stone,* 190 N.W. 2d 336 (Mich. 1971).
98. *Ebaugh v. Rankin, Cal. Rptr.* 99:706 (Cal. 1972).
99. *Black v. Caruso, Cal. Rptr.* 9:634 (Cal. 1960).
100. *Morse v. Moretti,* 403 F. 2d 564 (C.A. D.C. 1968).
101. *McBride v. Roy,* 58 P. 2d 886 (Okla. 1936).
102. *Mayo v. McClung,* 64 S.E. 2nd 330 (Ga. 1951).
103. *Barham v. Widing,* 291 Pac. 173 (Cal. 1930).
104. *Brown v. Hughes,* 30 P. 2d 259 (Colo. 1934).
105. *Haven v. Randolph,* 342 F. Supp. 538 (D.C. D.C. 1972).
106. *Shetler v. Rochelle,* 409 P. 2d 74 (Ariz. 1965).
107. *Miller v. Kennedy,* 522 P. 2d 852 (Wash. 1974).
108. Katz, J. Informed consent in the therapeutic relationship: Medical and legal aspects. In: *Encyclopedia of Bioethics.* Warren Reich, ed. Washington, D.C.: Georgetown University (in press).

109. *Canterbury v. Spence,* 464 F. 2d 772 (C.A. D.C. 1972).
110. Comment: The minor's right to abortion and the requirement of parental consent. *Va. Law Rev.,* 60(2):304, 1974.
111. *Baird v. Bellotti,* 393 F. Supp. 847 at 850 (D.C. Mass.).
112. *Bellotti v. Baird,* 424 U.S., 49 L. Ed. 2d 844, (1976).
113. *In re Anonymous,* 248 N.Y.S. 2d 608 (N.Y. 1964).
114. Ellis, J.W. Volunteering children: Parental commitment of minors to mental institutions. *Cal. Law Rev.,* 62:840, 1974.
115. *In re G, Cal. Rptr.* 104:585 (Cal. 1972).
116. Lessem, L. On the voluntary admission of minors. *U. Mich. J. Law Ref.,* 8:189, Fall, 1974.
117. *In re Sippy,* 97 A. 2d 455 (D.C. Mun. Ct. 1953).
118. Curran, W.J., and Beecher, H.K. Experimentation in children. *JAMA* 210(1):77, Oct. 6, 1969.
119. American Academy of Pediatrics. Drug testing in children: F.D.A. regulations. *Pediatrics,* 43(3):463, March, 1969.
120. Chalkley, D.T. *Medical World News,* p. 41, June 8, 1973.
121. Ramsey, P. *The Patient as Person.* New haven: Yale University Press, 1970.
122. McCormick, R.A. Proxy consent in the experimental situation. *Perspect. Biol. Med.,* 18(1):2, Autumn, 1974.
123. Capron, A.M. Legal considerations affecting clinical pharmacological studies in children. *Clin. Res.,* 21:141, Feb., 1973.
124. Lowe, C., Alexander, D., and Mishkin, B. Nontherapeutic research on children: An ethical dilemma. *J. Pediatrics,* 84(4):468, April, 1974.
125. *McKinnon v. First National Bank of Pensacola,* 82 So. 248 (Fla. 1919).
126. Levine, R.J. Appropriate guidelines for the selection of human subjects for participation in biomedical and behavioral research. Prepared for the National Commission for the Protection of Human Subjects of Biomedical and Behavioral Research, 1976.
127. Schoolar, J.C. and Gaitz, C.M., eds. *Research and the Psychiatric Patient.* New York: Brunner/Mazel, 1975.
128. Opinion 74-1675, Nov. 14, 1974. Attorney General of Louisiana.
129. *Burnham v. Department of Public Health of Georgia,* 394 F. Supp. 1335 (N.D. Ga. Aug. 3, 1972).
130. Kumasaka, Y., Stolles, J., and Gupta, R.K. Criteria for involuntary hospitalization. *Arch. Gen. Psychiat.,* 26:399-404, 1972.
131. Chodoff, P. The case for involuntary hospitalization of the mentally ill. *Amer. J. Psychiat.,* 133:496-501, 1976.
132. *Jacobson v. Massachusetts,* 197 U.S. 11 (1904).
133. *McGuire v. Amyx,* 217 No. 1061, 297 S.V. 968 (1927).
134. Murphy, J.N. Psychiatric labeling in cultural prospective. *Science,* 191:1019-1028, 1976.
135. May, P.R.A. Psychotherapy research in schizophrenia—Another view of present reality. *Schizophrenia Bull.,* pp. 126-132, 1974.
136. Stone, A.A. Overview: The right to treatment—Comments on the law and its impact. *Amer. J. Psychiat.,* 132:1125-1134, 1975.
137. Katz, J. The right to treatment: An enchanting legal fiction. *Univ. of Chicago L. Rev.* 36:755-783, 1969.
138. Federal Register-DHEW-PHS. Protection of human subjects: Policies and procedures. Vol. 39(105), May 30, 1974.

139. Olin, G.B., and Olin, H.S. Informed consent in voluntary mental hospital admissions. *Amer. J. Psychiat.*, 132:938-941, 1975.

140. Palmar, A.B., and Wohl, J. Voluntary admissions forms: Does the patient know what he is signing? *Hosp. Comm. Psychiat.*, 23:250-252, 1972.

141. Culleton, B.J. Confidentiality: Court declares researcher can protect sources. *Science*, 193:467-469, 1976.

142. Federal Register-DHEW-PHS. Confidentiality of alcohol and drug abuse patient records. Vol. 40(127), July, 1976.

143. Ennis, B.S. legal rights of the voluntary patient. *NAPPH Journ.*, 8:4-8, 1976.

144. Stone, B. ABA backs liability law changes. *Amer. Med. News*, Aug. 23, 1976.

145. Sciences. *N.Y. Acad. Science J.*, p. 5, Nov., 1976.

146. *Miranda v. Arizona*, 384 U.S. 436 (1966).

147. Spiotto, J. Search and seizure: An empirical study of the exclusionary rule and its alternatives. *J. Leg. Studies*, 2:243, 1973.

148. Oaks, D. Studying the exclusionary rule in search and seizure. *U. Chicago Law Rev.*, 37:665, 1970.

149. Spiller, D. *After Decision: Implementation of Judicial Decrees in Correctional Settings. A Case Study of Hamilton v. Schiro.* American Bar Foundation, 1976.

150. *Gagnon v. Scarpelli*, 411 U.S. 778 (1973).

151. *Morrissey v. Brewer*, 408 U.S. 471 (1972).

152. *Bell v. Burson*, 402 U.S. 535 (1971).

153. Force, R. *Procedural Due Process Requirements in Administrative Suspension and Revocations of Driver's Licenses.* (in press)

154. *Holt v. Sarver*, 300 F. Supp. 825 (E.D. Ark. 1969), 309 F. Supp. 362 (E.D. Ark. 1970), *aff'd.* 442 F. 2d 304 (8th Cir. 1971).

CHAPTER III

Research and the Law: Barriers and Progress

NEIL L. CHAYET

The last several years have been difficult ones for the researcher and the clinician. These years have seen a steady demand for the alleviation of disease, but a corresponding decline in the availability of the tools with which the researcher and the clinician can bring about this goal. The medical and scientific communities have become trapped, on the one hand, by the public's call for more and better care, and on the other, by the raising of barriers to the giving of that care in legislatures, courts, and regulatory agencies throughout the country. It may be that only a major coordinated effort can restore the ability of the scientist, researcher, and clinician to once again move toward the conquering of diseases such as schizophrenia and other major disorders that afflict thousands of human beings in this country and throughout the world.

This chapter will analyze the current legal barriers which have been erected in the path of the researcher, as well as his clinical brethren, since the problems faced by both have common threads. It will look at the many failures of the law in its attempt to regulate the research community, as well as its few successes. Lastly, it will attempt to map out a path for the future. It is written with the hope that the years ahead will bring a renaissance of research and a more hospitable relation between the law and the scientist and clinician.

The present difficulties have manifested themselves in a plethora of activities in the courts, the Congress, state legislatures, and federal and state regulatory agencies. It must be recognized, however, that these agencies, for the most part, reflect public opinion. The scientific and research communities must face the fact that large segments of the public do not understand the nature of the work done by the scientist in general and the biomedical researcher in particular. The public has been led to believe, through a series of occurrences, that the biomedical researcher and the clinician are not competent guardians of the rights of the individual. Governmental action has thus been deemed necessary to protect the rights of persons. Those judges, regulators, and legislators, for the most part, bear no malice toward the researcher, but simply are not cognizant of the futility of the regulatory process upon which they have embarked. It is the premise of this chapter that research and clinical efforts to alleviate suffering and disease and to prolong life have been greatly hampered by these various juridical, legislative, and other regulatory processes, and that the resultant protection of human subjects has not been materially improved over prior practices of researchers. When one considers that individuals and not society suffer from diseases such as schizophrenia, the present regulatory scheme must be viewed as a net loss for such individuals and for society as a whole.

It is unfortunate indeed that the work of the research community has been placed in contraposition to the fundamental rights and dignity of the individual. One might argue, on the contrary, that scientific inquiry is nurtured by the rights and dignity of the individual, that one of the most fundamental rights is that of being as free of debilitating mental and physical diseases as is humanly achievable, and that such freedom can only be preserved and furthered by intensive biomedical research into diseases such as schizophrenia which have remained thus far a mystery. It seems that only through scientific inquiry can we find the answers to the problems of alcoholism, drug abuse, and uncontrolled violent behavior, as we have found the answers to polio and plague.

Nevertheless, in November 1974, a sobering report was released by the Committee on the Judiciary, entitled "Individual Rights and the Federal Role in Behavior Modification" (1). The study was prepared by the staff of the Subcommittee on Constitutional Rights, chaired at that time by Senator Sam Ervin, a hero to those who believe in the importance of protecting fundamental human and constitutional rights. The tone of this report is set by the following segment:

> To my mind the most serious threat posed by the technology of behaviour modification is the power this technology gives one man to impose his views and values on another. In our democratic society values such as political and religious preferences are expressly left to individual choice.

If our society is to remain free, one man must not be empowered to change another man's personality and dictate the values, thoughts and feelings of another.

To begin with, there is the quest to advance scientific knowledge through experimentation which must be reconciled with our society's belief in the inviolability of a person's mind and body. Moreover, this personal autonomy must be reconciled with the need in certain circumstances for the state to restrict the individual's choice concerning experimental medical procedures in order to enhance or protect his autonomy and welfare.

The problem of ethical experimentation is the product of the unresolved conflict between two strongly held values: the dignity and integrity of the individual, and the freedom of scientific inquiry. Professionals of many disciplines, and researchers especially, exercise unexamined discretion to interfere in the lives of their subjects for the sake of scientific progress. Although exposure to needless harm and neglect of the duty to obtain the subject's consent have been generally frowned upon in theory, the infliction of unnecessary harm and infringements on informed consent are frequently accepted in practice as the price to be paid for the advancement of knowledge. How have investigators come to claim this sweeping prerogative? If the answer to this question is that society has authorized professionals to choose between scientific progress and individual human dignity and welfare, should not "society" retain some control over the research enterprise? We agree with Dr. Jonas that "a slower progress in the conquest of disease would not threaten society, grievous as it is to those who have to deplore that their particular disease be not yet conquered, but that society would indeed be threatened by the erosion of those moral values whose loss, possibly caused by too ruthless a pursuit of scientific progress, would make its most dazzling triumphs not worth having."

I am not saying that researchers should carry on their work with abandon, conscious only of the goal they seek and oblivious to the rights, dignity, and concerns of their subjects. Nor am I implying that there have been no abuses through the years. The Tuskegee study—a federally sponsored research program—was an exercise in both naiveté and reckless investigation. This incident has served as a major catalyst to restriction on research, just as the thalidomide incident resulted in the Kefauver legislation which, while providing many needed reforms, dealt a severe blow to new drug research and approval.

The distrust of the research effort has manifested itself in many ways— some blatant, some subtle—and all are equally destructive. The National Institute of Health (NIH) budget for the fiscal year 1975 was cut 1.6 billion dollars. But the vagaries of the budgetary process are well known and predictable, and reversible if the appropriate political pressure exists and is applied. Not so easily reversed or even understood are the themes that have been played out in the courts, in Congress, in federal and state regulatory agencies, and in state legislatures throughout the country.

THE COURTS

Two themes have been played out concurrently in the courts in recent years, with resultant destructiveness and a definite chilling of the research effort. These themes are: (a) the legal efforts on behalf of the institutionalized mentally ill; and (b) the common law development of the doctrine of informed consent.

The last decade has seen much activity on the part of those who have purported to represent the interests of the institutionalized mentally ill. During the mid-1960s and the early 1970s, the emphasis was on release of the institutionalized mentally ill. There is little question that there were severely abused procedures governing the commitment of the mentally ill, but some have wondered whether the premium placed on release of those commited was proper and whether the procurement of same was the most appropriate battle to be waged. I recall my own involvement in the civil libertarian efforts of the mid-1960s, and one case in particular stands out as representative of the difficulties in this area.

The case involved a fruit peddlar in Boston's North End who decided that business might improve if he made his horse more like a zebra. So he painted white stripes on the animal, was promptly arrested by the Boston police for the crime of defacing an animal, and was removed for observation to Bridgewater State Hospital for the criminally insane on the recommendation of the police. He had no attorney and did not even appear before a judge.

The doctors reported back to the court that the man was incompetent to stand trial; it was clear that they had not even understood the nature of the legal test to determine incompetency for trial. (Does the individual understand the crime with which he is charged, does he understand the nature of his relation to the crime, and is he able to cooperate with his attorney in his defense?) The individual involved was branded as incompetent for trial because they found he was "ill." This was in 1920; we discovered him at Bridgewater in 1967, and he died there in 1968, being most reluctant to leave the institution to which he had become very much accustomed over the course of forty years.

It is little wonder that many attorneys and others who cared about the civil rights of the mentally ill were incensed and took action to bring about the release of thousands of institutionalized mentally ill persons across the country. It became immediately apparent, however, that the mere release of institutionalized individuals back into the community was not an ultimate solution. I remember one individual who was arrested for simple assault in 1940 and whom I had released back to his community in 1967. A few months after his release, I began receiving regular calls from his brother who asked how much it would cost to have his brother recommitted. It seems that the man had done little since his release other than to ask to borrow money and be helped in getting a job.

In addition, some courts were becoming reluctant to release individuals who were deemed dangerous. Thus, in the late 1960s, another trend became evident. The cases marking this trend were inappropriately known as the "right-to-treatment" cases. Although billed as cases setting forth a constitutional right to treatment, they merely guaranteed a certain basic personal dignity and humane living conditions. Cases such as *Wyatt v. Stickney* (2) sought to somehow rectify the plight of patients in state mental institutions who had been subjected to intolerable living conditions. They were not, however, cases that gave a right to treatment, largely because it was not known, and still is not known, how such patients should be treated to alleviate or end their illness. If anything, these cases made it difficult to treat patients, for they marked the beginning of a trend which was to become very destructive a few years later—the intimation that persons of diminished capacity could not give consent for research projects, even those that were closely related to the disease from which they suffered. In *Wyatt v. Stickney* it was stated: "Patients shall have a right not to be subjected to experimental research without the express and informed consent of the patient, if the patient is able to give such consent, and of his guardian or next of kin, after opportunities for consultation with independent specialists and with legal counsel" (2).

This line of cases culminated with the recently decided case of *Donaldson v. O'Connor* (3) that held that a person must be released if he is not accorded proper "treatment." "Lack of treatment" in this case appeared, in reality, to be relegating Mr. Donaldson to mere custodial care. It is also relevant to note that this case fastened civil liability on the physician involved, who had failed to give the patient proper treatment.

While the courts throughout the country were speaking in terms of a mandated right to treatment, other lawyers were at work establishing what, in effect, prevented proper treatment, again in the name of protecting the rights of the mentally ill—a theme that was becoming widely utilized. The best known of these cases is *Kaimowitz v. Department of Mental Health of the State of Michigan* (4). The case dealt with psychosurgery and presented an unfortunate set of facts, proving the truth of the adage, "Hard cases make bad law." The court in the *Kaimowitz* case noted that there are three basic elements of informed consent: competency of the individual, knowledge of the risks, and voluntariness. In the case of an institutionalized mentally ill person, these three elements "cannot be ascertained with a degree of reliability" even by the physician, and thus the procedure was prohibited (4). It is important to emphasize that this case involved an irreversible invasive procedure, but it is clear that this case was but the beginning of a deliberate attempt to halt all research with institutionalized mentally ill individuals. Following the *Kaimowitz* decision, the same attorney sought in *Jobes et al. v. Michigan Department of Mental Health* (5) to prevent the administration of zinc to children as part of a research project. While this did not succeed, it is clear that we have not seen the end of the cases that stand for a right to no treatment and that make it impossible to perform the research that may, in fact, lead to appropriate treatment.

In summary, it is difficult to assess the net result of the considerable work of those who have labored for the civil liberties of the mentally ill. It has now become virtually impossible to commit persons unless there is clear proof of their dangerousness. This is probably a significant improvement over the past, but there is little question that many persons who are in need of treatment are untreated, barely existing in apathetic or hostile communities. Those who are institutionalized are probably receiving a higher level of care, at least in terms of their physical surroundings. But as for research and treatment with regard to the disease process that caused their hospitalization, little progress is being made, and it can be said that the law is now actively intervening to prevent further progress toward the conquest of their disease.

A second theme related to the above trends is the development of a body of case law defining informed consent in increasingly restrictive terms and applying such definitions to the mentally disabled in a manner that will make it virtually impossible for research to be carried on with such individuals. Briefly stated, the fundamental principle at issue is that if a person is going to receive treatment or participate in a research project, he must give his consent to do so. Such consent must be based on an understanding of the procedure and its risks and benefits to the person involved.

Most of the case law in the area of informed consent has come from medical and dental malpractice cases. It is of interest to note that the earliest malpractice case on record concerned human experimentation in which the defendant doctor used an unconventional method in treating a leg fracture with a poor result: "The defendant Baker put on to the plaintiff's leg an heavy steel thing that had teeth . . . and broke the leg again, and three or four months afterward the plaintiff was still very ill. It seems as if Mr. Baker wanted to try an experiment with this new instrument" (6).

The clearest examples of failure to obtain informed consent may be found in those classic cases in which the wrong tooth is extracted or the wrong limb is removed or operated on (for instance, *Mohr v. Williams* [7] where the wrong ear was operated on). The skill with which the procedure is performed is irrelevant, since all that need be shown is that the patient did not consent. The only universal exception to the rule requiring informed consent has been in the giving of emergency care (8). From a legal perspective, the concept of informed consent is a sound one, but many lawyers, judges, and regulators fail to appreciate the difficulties encountered in securing informed consent from patients who are mentally disabled or even from those persons who are facing serious medical or surgical procedures.

The basic questions that have caused so much difficulty are: What constitutes proper consent? Who are the appropriate persons from whom it has to be secured? And assuming that informed consent has been properly secured from the appropriate person, how does one go about proving that fact in litigation that may occur many years subsequent to the event?

For the most part, the basic ingredients appear to be the indication of a willingness to have a procedure performed after an explanation and understanding of the procedure and the risks and benefits associated with it. There is much controversy as to which risks have to be described. Some courts have required that virtually all risks be detailed for the patient, regardless of the impact that this policy of full disclosure may have on the patient. Other courts have sought to allow the measurement of a community standard of care; that is, what would the average prudent physician or researcher in the community have told the patient? This standard implies permitting the physician to take into account the psychological impact of the information on the patient and to tailor the information given to the ability of the patient to understand and appreciate, and not be harmed by, the information. The most often quoted reference to the concept that gives credence to the psychological needs of the patient is the Helsinki declaration, which provides: "If at all possible, consistent with patient psychology, the doctor should obtain the patient's freely given consent after the patient has been given a full explanation" (9).

The major problem is that a full statement of all or even the major risks of a procedure will very often have a serious, adverse psychological effect on a patient or a research subject. This is true with a "normal" patient or subject; it becomes particularly attenuated and often impossible when the patient is mentally disabled or otherwise impaired.

The clinician's or researcher's concern about the question of informed consent will not be diminished by a rather bizarre Connecticut case (as yet unreported formally) of a patient who visited a physician to discuss his forthcoming coronary-bypass operation. The physician, who had become extremely concerned about being sued and who thought that this patient might prove to be rather litigious, decided to take extraordinary precautions and, in minute detail, informed the frightened patient of all the potential risks of coronary-bypass surgery. The patient, after listening for a while, became paler and paler and finally left the doctor's office, refusing to continue the conversation or to undergo the surgery. He returned home and died a short time later. Suit has been brought against the physician for wrongfully causing the death of the patient by the manner in which he sought to secure the patient's informed consent.

Even if informed consent is obtained, and bypassing for the moment the question of whom it has to be obtained from, there are major problems in the manner in which the informed consent is documented so that it may be proved in later years. The traditional method of documentation is by way of a form that is signed by the patient and may or may not be witnessed. Another method is a notation by the physician on the patient's chart. These methods are not without hazard. The notation on the chart is subject to the later claim that it was little more than a routine, self-serving statement; even the signed form is subject to later claims of misunderstanding, incompetence, or duress. Witnesses to these documents may be subject to attack on the basis of bias if employed by the physician or researcher whose acts are under question. Some physicians, in desperation, have begun taping all patient interviews when informed consent is being secured, and at least one is considering videotaping the session!

The problems surrounding informed consent become particularly acute when one is dealing with the mentally disabled, especially in the research setting. Under the laws of virtually all jurisdictions, a person is legally competent to give consent or to take any legal action, unless declared legally incompetent by a court of appropriate jurisdiction. The fact of a person's commitment or institutionalization does not, in and of itself, render that person legally incompetent. However, as a practical matter, it is often the case that an individual who is in an institution, while perhaps legally competent, does not have the ability to understand what is being explained to him or her, and therefore the nature of the consent secured is severely tainted. And we have already seen that there is at least one case, *Kaimowitz* (4), that, regardless of the question of legal competency, holds that an institutionalized mentally disabled person is incapable of giving informed consent for a research project.

Some have met with partial success in their attempts to avoid difficulty. In Kentucky, the state court in *Strunk v. Strunk* authorized a transplant operation to be performed with a mentally incompetent patient as the donor by utilizing the legal doctrine of substituted judgment. Since the incompetent was unable to exercise his competent judgment, the court substituted its own judgment (10). An analogy can be drawn in the situation wherein consent is required to perform an operation on a minor. In the case of *Bonner v. Moran* (11), the court found the consent of a parent to be legally sufficient, even if the operation has no direct therapeutic value for the child.

In Louisiana, the current law, as stated in *In re Richardson* (12), does not permit the guardian of an incompetent to utilize his judgment in the incompetent's best interests. However, a researcher was able to secure an opinion of the Attorney General for the State of Louisiana to the effect that next of kin could legally consent to an institutionally committed relative's participation in a research project. While attorney generals' opinions are not binding on actions that may subsequently be taken by a court, they are useful and may well be dispositive of the manner in which a court will deal with the question when a specific challenge is made.

Others have suggested that a guardian be appointed for the mentally ill person, implying that this is the solution to all difficulties. In one state, a probate judge habitually appointed an attorney guardian for mentally disabled persons placed in an institution under the court's jurisdiction. This attorney, without ever even seeing his wards, would routinely consent to their participation in research projects that were placed before him for signature. He did so because he had great confidence in the researcher, but little need be said about the problems that would result if such a *pro forma* procedure was ever challenged. In general, it is virtually impossible to have a guardian appointed, even for the limited purpose of approving participation in a research project. The reason is that lawyers, family members, and others who usually become guardians are extermely reluctant to take on the responsibility of having consented to such a procedure; moreover, many are simply not available since there is no prospect of compensation in most of these cases. In addition, the appointment of a guardian is often a complicated procedure that requires the filing of petitions, inventories, and the like.

CRIMINAL LEGISLATION

A third theme, and perhaps the most disturbing of all for the researcher, is the increasing application of the criminal law to this area. One of the most celebrated cases involved four researchers at Boston City Hospital who attempted to ascertain which drugs were most successful in the treatment of certain congenital diseases. Women who had come to the hospital for voluntary abortions gave their informed consent to participate in a study in which they would take an antibiotic or a control agent prior to the abortion, and the fetal tissue would be studied following the abortion to ascertain the effectiveness of the drugs used. The resultant study was published in the *New England Journal of Medicine* (13), and this precipitated the indictment of the four physicians involved for the crime of graverobbing. The pertinent statute (14) reads as follows:

> Whoever, not being lawfully authorized by the proper authorities, willfully digs up, disinters, removes or conveys away a human body, or the

remains thereof, or knowingly aids in such disinterment, removal or con-
veying away, and whoever is accessory thereto either before or after the
fact shall be punished by imprisonment in the state prison for not more
than two and one half years or by a fine of not more than two thousand
dollars.

This case, which is still awaiting trial in Massachusetts, has resulted in a
statute which makes it a criminal offense to do research with fetuses slated
for abortion. Thus, research can only be done with those fetuses not planned for abortion (15). The reason, as stated by one proponent of the legislation, is that the only way to protect all fetuses, including those that are to
be aborted is to require that only fetuses that are not going to be aborted
could be the subjects of research projects. As originally drafted, the
law cast doubt on whether or not amniocentesis could be performed. The
statute was subsequently clarified to permit such research when the life or
health of the particular fetus was involved.

The above legislation became the subject of intense lobbying by researchers, who received a great deal of meaningful assistance with their efforts from
groups such as the Tay-Sachs Foundation and other groups dedicated to the
prevention and early detection of congenital diseases. The mothers involved
in one organization descended en masse on the State House and crowded into
meeting rooms in the Governor's office, legislative halls, and all other places
where the bill was under discussion. One mother testified most effectively.
She had had a child who was born with and died from Tay-Sachs disease.
She then became pregnant again and through amniocentesis learned that her
second baby could have this dread disease, and she aborted that fetus. But
amniocentesis also proved that her third pregnancy would result in a normal
child, and she gave her testimony while holding this child in her arms. This
experience shows the importance of forming new coalitions between those
who carry out the research and those who benefit from it.

There has been additional difficulty in the area of informed consent. One
individual in Massachusetts was convicted of carrying out a research project
without securing the informed consent of a subject who subsequently died,
although it was never proven that the death of the subject was in any way
connected with the research project. The statute under which the researcher
was convicted provides for criminal penalties for failure to obtain informed
consent (16).

REGULATORY AGENCIES

What is most unfortunate is that a certain degree of competitiveness
seems to have evolved with regard to the activities of various agencies. This

spirit of competitive control seems to be most evident within the Department of Health, Education, and Welfare (DHEW) which has taken extremely aggressive action resulting in serious problems for the researchers, again, without concomitant improvement in the protection of human subjects.

Present regulations require an Institutional Review Board (IRB) and also require that the subject or his legally authorized representative give informed consent for involvement in any research project (17). There is little question that the establishment of IRBs has led to significant improvement in the manner in which research projects are carried on in institutions throughout the United States. The presence of individuals who are neither involved in the research project nor even, in some cases, with the institution has been a helpful development in dealing with the ethical issues involved in research. It is clear that protocols themselves have often been significantly improved by exposure to an IRB. The present difficulties with the IRB are the manner in which it is organized and the mandated presence of a large number of non-institutional persons. In Massachusetts, for example, many of the presently constituted IRBs are illegal because they do not have the requisite number of community representatives. In other words, the problem is not with the IRB concept itself, but with the manner in which this process is being altered, restricted, and encumbered by federal and state regulatory and legislative activity.

Proposed federal regulations (18) would greatly hamper the existing process by requiring the establishment of an Organizational Review Committee (ORC) to ensure that research subjects have not received undue inducements to participate in the experiment and to protect the confidentiality of the subject and the results of any research. Such a committee would also be charged with assuring that the selection procedures are adequate.

In addition, the proposed regulations require that a Consent Committee (CC) be established to assure that legally effective consent has been obtained. This committee would also be charged with monitoring the activities and the continued willingness of the subjects to participate, conducting site visits, and intervening on behalf of the subjects if conditions warrant it. Such a committee would "have the authority to terminate participation of one or more subjects with or without their consent, where conditions warrant" (19).

The problem with all of this is that there are simply not enough people available to serve on the committees that presently exist. Also, there have been a number of law suits, and there is concern that the potential liability of persons who serve on these committees will dissuade many from serving.

Perhaps the most acute problems exist in the area of informed consent, with a peculiar, paralyzing paradox having been created by the activities of different federal agencies within the DHEW. Regulations of the Food and Drug Administration (FDA) require well-controlled clinical studies that depend on the ability of researchers to secure research subjects to carry out such studies (20). The paradox is, however, that regulations of both the FDA itself and other agencies within the DHEW have made it increasingly difficult to secure such subjects and, in many contexts, securing them has become impossible. For example, many of the well-controlled clinical trials were carried on by drug companies in prisons, and recent promulgations have placed serious restrictions on prison research.

The Food, Drug and Cosmetic Act provides that clinical investigators shall "obtain the consent of such human beings or their representatives, except where they deem it not feasible or, in their professional judgment, contrary to the best interests of such human beings" (21). In conducting clinical research using investigational new drugs (INDs), FDA regulations require that the sponsor obtain a signed statement from each investigator which contains assurances from IRBs that the investigator has obtained the informed consent of the human subjects, *except where it has not been feasible to do so or where it would be contrary to the best interests of those subjects.* Failure to comply with these requirements would disqualify the investigator from receiving INDs, and the Commission may disapprove a New Drug Application (NDA) if the sponsor's "notice of claimed investigational exemption" contains data from an ineligible investigator (22).

The problem with the requirements of the FDA regulations, although they are far more liberal than those involved in DHEW-funded studies, is that the regulations would probably not withstand a legal challenge. The researcher faces potential liability if he were, for example, to proceed to carry out research on incompetent individuals after having deemed the securing of informed consent unfeasible merely because the research subjects were totally incompetent. The state statutory and regulatory requirements, including the prospect of criminal liability under some statutes looked at above, would operate to greatly discourage such activity, to say nothing of the civil liability that would probably result as in the cases discussed above.

The conflict becomes even clearer when one looks at the current DHEW regulations governing informed consent in biomedical and behavioral research. These regulations set forth a federal standard for informed consent that is defined as follows:

> ... the knowing consent of an individual or his legally authorized representative, so situated as to be able to exercise free power of choice without undue inducement or any element of force, fraud, deceit, duress, or other form of constraint or coercion. The basic elements of information necessary to such consent include:
>
> (1) A fair explanation of the procedures to be followed, and their purposes, including identification of any procedures which are experimental;

(2) A description of any attendant discomforts and risks reasonably to be expected;

(3) A description of any benefits reasonably to be expected;

(4) A disclosure of any appropriate alternative procedures that might be advantageous for the subject;

(5) An offer to answer any inquiries concerning the procedures; and

(6) An instruction that the person is free to withdraw his consent and to discontinue participation in the project or activity at any time without prejudice to the subject [23].

An analysis of these regulations indicates that while there will be some situations where it is possible to obtain the informed consent of institutionalized individuals, there will be many cases where it is impossible, practically and legally, to obtain such consent because of the limited capacity of the individuals involved. And, as stated above, there is great difficulty in coming up with legally authorized representatives, whose appointments are usually governed by the vagaries of state law. Most states presently require the appointments of guardians or conservators, but this is extremely difficult and virtually impossible in most situations. The definition of "legally authorized representative" is as follows: ". . . an individual or judicial or other body authorized under applicable law to consent on behalf of a prospective subject to such subject's participation in the particular activity or procedure" (24).

Following the passage of the National Research Act in 1974 (P.L. 93-348), the DHEW proposed additional regulations designed to provide further protective measures for those subjects of research whose capability of providing informed consent may be absent or limited. These subjects included children, pregnant women, fetuses, prisoners, and the mentally disabled. The mentally disabled are defined in these proposed regulations as those who are mentally ill, retarded, emotionally disturbed, and confined either voluntarily or involuntarily. It is of interest to note that the courts have relied on the policy evinced by P.L. 93-348 to support at least one plaintiff's claim for relief as the subject of alleged "inhumane treatment."

The issue in the case of *Clay v. Martin* (25) was whether the plaintiff's allegation of "inhumane treatment" while a federal prisoner was sufficient to state a claim which would entitle him to relief if proved. The plaintiff claimed that he was a participant in an experiment in which he was administered Naltrexone, a drug thought to prevent narcotics from exhibiting euphoric or dependency effects. The plaintiff alleged further that the physician in charge told him that the dosage was too small to cause any harm, but he claimed that, as a result of the administration of the drug, he suffered a serious heart attack. Citing P.L. 93-348, the court said, "The legislative history of the Act indicates that it was passed in reaction to reports of abuses similar to those alleged here . . . in view of these expressions of public policy a court should not be quick to dismiss on pleading technicalities an action involving experimentation on humans" (25).

Most disturbing is language in the proposed regulations that could result in a total ban on any research with the institutionalized mentally ill, a goal that may well be in the minds of some of the writers of these regulations. The regulations (26) provide:

Sec. 46.503 Activities involving the institutionalized mentally disabled.

Institutionalized mentally disabled individuals may not be included in an activity covered by this subpart unless:

(a) The proposed activity is related to the etiology, pathogenesis, prevention, diagnosis, or treatment of mental disability or the management, training, or rehabilitation of the mentally disabled and seeks information which cannot be obtained from subjects who are not institutionalized mentally disabled;

(b) The individual's legally effective informed consent to participation in the activity or, where the individual is legally incompetent, the informed consent of a representative with legal authority so to consent on behalf of the individual has been obtained; and

(c) The individual's assent to such participation has also been secured, when in the judgment of the consent committee he or she has sufficient mental capacity to understand what is proposed and to express an opinion as to his or her participation.

It is unclear from these regulations how one proves that the information sought in the research "cannot be obtained from subjects who are not institutionalized mentally disabled." Nor is it clear how one shows that the proposed activity is related to the condition from which the individual is suffering and what threshold of assurance is indicated.

The proposed regulations contain the same ambiguities with regard to informed consent as do the present regulations, with one significant addition:

(b) Nothing in this subpart shall be construed as indicating that compliance with the procedures set forth herein will necessarily result in a legally effective consent under applicable State or local law to a subject's participation in such an activity; nor in particular does it obviate the need for court approval of such participation where court approval of such participation is required under applicable State or local law in order to obtain a legally effective consent [27].

This means that instead of taking the opportunity to establish a definitive federal policy with regard to the question of informed consent, the federal government has instead opted to leave the researcher—and the research subject, for that matter—to the vagaries of state law.

CONCLUSIONS AND RECOMMENDATIONS

It is important, as we approach the years ahead, to learn from the errors of the past and to at least not worsen the situation. One would hope that the governmental and judicial interventions of the past several years have shown us what not to do, even if these experiences have not shown us a clear path that should be followed. There are, however, a number of problems that may make a change in direction extremely difficult. The first of these is the very nature of government and bureaucracy. Once the bureaucracy invades a given field of interest, it is extremely difficult to dislodge it or persuade it to reduce its efforts. Those who are responsible for the drafting of regulations turn out an enormous amount of material, much of which is acknowledged to be unnecessary or irelevant; in turn, the various interest groups file comments which are of limited impact; and finally, in desperation, and if the stakes are high enough, there is the resort to action in the courts. The process is expensive, time-consuming, and often futile, since the courts, acting as the final arbiters, are becoming increasingly reluctant to make judgments on the merits of a case and prefer to act only when there is a procedural defect. What is most unfortunate is that, with few exceptions, the actors in this recurring drama believe that they are acting in the public interest; this being the case, it is extremely difficult to effect change or even to ascertain in which direction the public interest truly lies.

The challenge of the years ahead will be the intelligent dismantling of the bureaucracy and the realization that it is simply impossible to regulate everything. The question will be how to accomplish the goal of deregulation of that which cannot or should not be regulated by governmental intervention. The path to this goal will be a difficult one, but it may lie in the direction of the creation of different, and hopefully more exact, methods of control or behavior that will depend more on internalized controls exerted by professionals upon themselves than on constant and costly external intervention by governmental agencies.

At present, the future plans, insofar as they are known, are more of the past. There are plans for patient package inserts, more restrictive informed-consent guidelines, permanence for the National Commission for the Protection of Human Subjects of Biomedical and Behavioral Research (NCPHSBBR), additional committees within institutions, and there is even talk of reducing to writing all decisions by IRBs in an attempt to create a whole new body of "common law" in the area of research. There is also the possibility that criminal sanctions and penalties will be added as enforcement measures against researchers and clinicians, particularly in the areas of monitoring studies and the development of adverse drug reactions.

If one is to bring about change, it is necessary to engage the support of the natural constituencies who would benefit from and favor such change. It is clear that if we are to have any major successes over the next several years, it cannot be by acting alone. The public, the press, and the politicians are unhappy with many of the professions at the present time. There is an increasing spirit of anti-intellectualism and antiprofessionalism, and leading the list of those professions that currently make up political fodder are the scientists and the doctors, followed closely, by the way, by lawyers.

Those of us who seek change must join together, within and without. In the past, if something affected the clinician, the researcher paid little heed; even within disciplines, if something affected one group, e.g., the fetal researchers, the neuropsychopharmacologists paid only passing interest. We must realize that there are so many common enemies that without a solid internal front little progress will be made.

In addition, we must join with the ultimate beneficiaries of science and research—the public. The public must be shown that the true public interest lies not in the stifling of research and the proliferation of the bureaucracy, but in the encouragement of responsible research that will hopefully lead to the alleviation of the intense stress and anxiety that permeates all levels of life in the United States and throughout the world, and that will lead to conquering or mitigating the morbidity and mortality caused by physical and mental diseases that continue largely unabated. Somehow, we must make it politically popular to espouse research rather than to disparage it. We must also deal with a press that has had a destructive impact on science and research. The research community which, by and large, has heretofore interacted negatively with the press could alter the unfortunate biases of some members of the press through education and intensive work. Hopefully, the public will soon begin to wonder why we have not conquered certain diseases, why we have fewer new drugs, and why the products that do emerge are so costly. We must be ready with the answers, and work now to build the case that will show the destructiveness and the costs of the present regulatory system.

We must realize, however, that the scientific, research, and medical communities are not without their problems. It is fair to say that the scientific community has functioned largely as an elite group, paying relatively little heed to the needs of the people who are research subjects and the ultimate beneficiaries or consumers of the fruits of research. This is not to say that the incidence of actual harm to research subjects has been great. But the great publicity given to the Tuskeegee study and the Long Island cancer implant studies has been extraordinarily destructive—and even at that, the actual harm from what was done in these cases is not fully known. It is clear that there has been less than adequate communication between the research community and the public, and the aspect of paternalism has been a dominant theme that has angered many of those who find themselves taking action against the research community.

It will be futile and inappropriate to merely seek a return to "freedom" for the researcher. What is necessary is to ascertain what should be controlled and regulated and also to change the attitude of the public regarding the researcher.

A basic concern is the manner in which the researcher communicates with the research subject; also, a more functional system than the present one concerning informed consent is needed. One viable possibility for a more functional system lies in the presence of a third party who would, in essence, be able to fulfill the oft-lacking communication between the researcher and the subject. Such a person would be able to certify for legal purposes that the subject understood the risks and benefits of the research project. In the case of diminished capacity of the subject, this individual should have legal author- ity to consent on behalf of the subject. An appropriate title for this individual would be "patient surrogate," in order to avoid the concept implied by words such as "patient advocate."

With regard to attitudinal change, it is imperative to get across to the public that we do not live in a risk-free society and that medical and basic scientific progress can only be made with some risk and cost.

In summary, it is necessary to replace the present regulations with func- tional systems that bring about the goals sought for them and to influence the attitudes of the public and the press in a positive manner. The design of functional systems, the building of internal controls, and the changing of atti- tudes will not be an easy task, but must be accomplished if we are to main- tain and improve our efforts to alleviate suffering, to conquer disease, and to improve the quality of life.

COMMENTARIES

Terminological Inexactitude

DR. LEVINE: Rather than respond to each of Mr. Chayet's remarks that trouble me—and there are many of them—I shall suggest that there are some serious conceptual and semantic problems that tend to undermine most of our efforts to discuss the law as it relates to research. Since this is presented as a commentary on Mr. Chayet's paper, I should make it clear that neither he nor his profession should be blamed for the creation of these problems. Some of our most distinguished colleagues in biomedical research collaborated vigorously with lawyers, as well as various other professionals, in their de- velopment. Three of the more important problems are:

1. We fail to distinguish adequately between research, on the one hand, and the accepted and routine practice of medicine on the other. Because we fail to make these distinctions, we commonly find ourselves developing ethical norms, guidelines, and regulations that do not fit the class of activities for which they are designed.

2. We distinguish therapeutic from nontherapeutic research as if these were two distinct sets of activities and, further, as if the distinction—if it could be made—would be meaningful. This spurious dichotomization leads us to reach wrong conclusions in our ethical analyses and, as an inevitable consequence, to develop inappropriate law.

3. We tend to view research as a highly risky business and the role of research subject as a hazardous occupation. This incorrect assumption leads us to create highly complex mechanisms to protect human subjects from risk and then to apply them uniformly to all research activities, even though most present no risk of consequential physical or psychological harm. Further, this incorrect assumption tends to tarnish the public image of research.

The first three sections of this commentary will consist of an elaboration of the points made in the preceding paragraph. The fourth is a response to Mr. Chayet's remarks about the bureaucracy that is being developed in research institutions and to his proposed alternative—"the patient surrogate."

Distinctions between Research and Practice

At first glance, it might not seem difficult to most physicians to distinguish research from practice. And yet, in the legislative history of Title II of P.L. 93-348—the Act which created the National Commission for the Protection of Human Subjects of Biomedical and Behavioral Research (hereafter referred to as the Commission [NCPHSBBR])—we find that some most distinguished physicians regarded this as a very important and exceedingly difficult task (28, pp. 16-18). Jay Katz identified "drawing the line between research and accepted practice . . . [as] the most difficult and complex problem facing the Commission." Thomas Chalmers stated: "It is extremely hard to distinguish between clinical research and the practice of good medicine. Because episodes of illness and individual people are so variable, every physician is carrying out a small research project when he diagnoses and treats a patient."

Chalmers, of course, was only echoing the views of many distinguished physicians who had spoken to this issue earlier. For example, in *Experimentation with Human Subjects,* Herrman Blumgart (29) stated: "Every time a physician administers a drug to a patient, he is in a sense performing an experiment" (p. 44). To this Francis Moore (30) added that "every (surgical) operation of any type contains certain aspects of experimental work" (p. 358). While these statements are true, they tend to obfuscate the real issues; they tend to make more difficult the task of distinguishing research from practice.

What I am about to say represents something of a departure from what I have written earlier on the distinctions between research and practice (31, 32). My conception of these distinctions has evolved, in part, as a consequence of continuing discussions with the Commissioners of the NCPHSBBR, their consultants, and others. At this point I suggest that, as we consider the professional activities of physicians involving interactions with patients and/ or subjects, it would be most appropriate to classify these activities in four distinct sets. Definitions of the first three sets are taken from the Commission's draft of February 24, 1976, of "The boundaries between biomedical and behavioral research and accepted and routine practice." The fourth class of activities is defined in a paper that I prepared at the request of the Commission (33).

1. *Research:* "Biomedical and behavioral research involving human subjects refers to a class of activities designed to develop or contribute to generalizable knowledge. By generalizable knowledge we mean theories, principles or relationships (or the accumulation of data on which they may be based) that can be corroborated by accepted scientific observation and inferences."

2. *Practice:* "By contrast, the practice of medicine or behavioral therapy refers to a class of activities designed solely to enhance the well-being of an individual. The customary standard for routine and accepted practice is a reasonable expectation of success. The absence of validation or precision on which to base such an expectation, however, does not in and of itself define the activity in question as research. Uncertainty is inherent in therapeutic practice because of the variability of physiological and behavioral human response. This kind of uncertainty is, itself, routine and accepted."

3. *Innovative therapy:* ". . . other uncertainties may be introduced by the application of novel procedures, as for example, when deviations from common practice in drug administration or in surgical, medical or behavioral therapies are tried in the course of rendering treatment. These activities may be designated innovative therapy, but they do not constitute research unless formally structured as a research project . . . there is concern that innovative therapies are being applied in an unsupervised way, as part of practice. It is our recommendation that significant innovations in therapy *should* be incorporated into a research project in order to establish their safety and efficacy while retaining the therapeutic objectives."

It is made clear in other parts of this draft that diagnostic and prophylactic maneuvers are included under this rubric. Thus, a more descriptive title for this class of activities might be "innovative practices" (31). In subsequent discussion in more recent meetings of the Commission, it has become apparent that novelty is not the attribute that defines this class of practices; rather, it is the lack of suitable validation of the safety or efficacy of the practice. I therefore propose that the best designation for this class of activities is "nonvalidated practice." A practice might be nonvalidated because it is new, i.e., it has not been tested sufficiently often or sufficiently well to permit a satisfactory prediction of its safety or efficacy in a patient population. An equally common way for a practice to merit the designation "nonvalidated" is that in the course of its use in the practice of medicine there arises some legitimate cause to question previously held assumptions about its safety and/or efficacy. This might be because the practice was never validated adequately in the first place (e.g., implantation of the internal mammary artery for the treatment of coronary artery disease, treatment of gastric ulcers with antacids, treatment of cholera with turpentine stupes); because a question arises of a previously unknown serious toxicity (e.g., liver toxicity of iproniazid, renal failure with some sulfa preparations); or because a new practice seems likely to be either safer or more effective (e.g., replacement of arsenicals by penicillin). At the time of the first substantial challenge to the validity of a previously accepted practice, continuing use of that practice should be considered nonvalidated. For purposes of developing ethical norms, guidelines, or regulations, all nonvalidated practices may be considered together. As the Commission has suggested for innovative therapy, these practices should be conducted in the context of a research project designed to test their safety and efficacy; however, the research should not interfere with the basic therapeutic (or diagnostic or prophylactic) objectives.

4. *Practice for the benefit of others:* As we examine the universe of professional activities of physicians, we find that there is one set that does not conform to the definitions of research, practice, or nonvalidated practice. It departs from the definition of practice only in that it is not "designed solely to enhance the well-being of an individual." It does, however, meet "The customary standard for routine and accepted practice"—namely, "a reasonable expectation of success" (33, pp. 11-13). Thus, it does not conform to the definitions of either research, practice, or nonvalidated practice.

While the activities conducted in this category may bring direct health-related benefit to the patient, this is not necessarily the case. For example, one activity in this class—the donation of an organ (e.g., kidney) or tissue (e.g., blood)—brings no direct health benefit to the donor. Here the beneficiary is one other person who may or may not be related to the "patient." In some cases the beneficiary may be society generally as well as the individual patient (e.g., vaccination), while in others the only beneficiary may be society (e.g., quarantine). In some cases individuals are called upon to undergo psychosurgery, behavior modification, psychotherapy, or psychochemotherapy so as to be potentially less harmful to others; this is a particular problem when the individual is offered the "free choice" between the "sick role" and the "criminal role." In other cases the beneficiaries may include succeeding generations, as when patients are called upon to undergo sterilization because they are considered either genetically defective or otherwise incompetent to be parents; the problems in this area are illustrated in the discussion of the Relf case that figured importantly in the development of the congressional mandate to the Commission (28, pp. 26-28). In still other cases one beneficiary of the therapy may be an institution, and there may be serious disputes over the extent to which the purpose of therapy is to benefit the "patient" or to provide administrative convenience to the institution (e.g., heavy tranquilization of disruptive patients in a mental institution, treatment of hyperkinetic school-age children with various stimulant and depressive drugs).

What is the consequence of having identified a class of activities with the ungainly designation "practice for the benefit of others?" I have argued that it would be inappropriate to apply the ethical norms and guidelines developed for research to activities meeting the definition of medical practice (33). The main basis for my argument was that the rationale for the development of these norms and guidelines relates to certain attributes of research that do not exist in practice. One of the key distinctions is that in research the prospective subject is called upon to decide how much risk of physical, psychological, or other harm (or inconvenience) he or she will assume in exchange for benefits other than direct health-related benefits. These benefits might be economic (the subject might be paid), psychosocial (there might be an appeal to the subject's sense of altruism), and so on. In practice, on the other hand, almost all decisions may be based on a personal felicific calculus. The patient decides how much risk—usually based on statistics derived from previous experience—of physical or psychological harm he or she will assume for a statistically based expectation of physical or psychological benefit. In the category of practice for the benefit of others we tend to find the more complex "harm-benefit" analyses characteristic of research. It is these more complex analyses that provide the rationale for some of the procedures that are appropriate for research but not for practice. Thus, the four procedures designed to implement ethical norms developed to meet the needs of research might also be appropriate for some activities in the category of practice for the benefit of others. These are: (a) a meticulous description of the proposed activity in the form of a protocol; (b) review by an accountability structure analogous to the IRB prior to the initiation of the activity; (c) a high degree of formality in documenting the negotiations for informed consent; and (d) the development of a "no-fault" system of compensation for harmed patients (33).

Therapeutic vs. Nontherapeutic Research

It is not clear to me when this unfortunate distinction began to be made in discussions of the ethics and regulation of research. The Nuremberg Code (1947) makes no distinction (34). The Declaration of Helsinki (1964) distinguishes nontherapeutic clinical research from clinical research combined with professional care (9). In the 1975 revision of this Declaration, "medical research combined with professional care" is designated "clinical research" while "non-therapeutic biomedical research involving human subjects" is designated "non-clinical biomedical research." One major problem with this dichotomy is illustrated by placing a principle developed for clinical research (II.6) in immediate proximity to one developed for nonclinical research (III.2). "II.6: The doctor can combine medical research with professional care, the objective being the acquisition of new medical knowledge, only to the extent that medical research is jusitifed by its potential diagnostic or therapeutic value for the patient." "III.2: The subjects should be volunteers—either healthy persons or patients for whom the experimental design is not related to the patient's illness." In recent years, we have seen the distinction between therapeutic and nontherapeutic research assume a central position in the papers of those who discuss the ethics (35) or law (36) of research involving human subjects.

It is beyond the scope of my commentary to even list all of the problems that derive from the use of this unfortunate distinction. For the present purposes I shall confine my discussion to the identification of only three; these three are sufficiently serious that an awareness of them should force us to conclude that we must abandon this classification.

1. Many types of research done by physicians on human subjects cannot be defined as either therapeutic or nontherapeutic. Consider, for example, the placebo-controlled, "double-blind" drug trial. Certainly we cannot believe that the administration of a placebo for research purposes "is justified by its potential diagnostic or therapeutic value for the patient." Therefore, it is nontherapeutic. According to the Declaration of Helsinki, those who receive the placebo must be "either healthy persons or patients for whom the experimental design is not related to the patient's illness." This, of course, is absurd.

2. A strict interpretation of the Declaration of Helsinki would lead us to conclude that all rational research designed to explore the pathogenesis of a disease is to be forbidden. Since it cannot be justified as prescribed in Principle II.6, it must be considered nontherapeutic and therefore conducted only on healthy persons or patients not having the disease one wishes to investigate. Again, this is absurd.

3. Paul Ramsey provides us with a good example of how one can be led to erroneous conclusions by assuming that there is a distinction between therapeutic and nontherapeutic research (35, p. 11). He claims that the use of a nonconsenting subject is wrong, whether or not there is risk, simply because it involves an "unconsented touching." This wrongful touching is rectified only when it is for the good of the individual. Thus, based on the assumption that therapeutic research is always done for the good of the individual subject, he concludes that proxy consent is permissible for therapeutic research. He further concludes that nontherapeutic research on children is never justified because they cannot consent for themselves and the "good" that would validate proxy consent to therapeutic research is lacking.

In order to avoid these embarrassments, we must abandon the distinction between therapeutic and nontherapeutic research. The definition of research that we should use is the one developed by the Commission cited above. Sometimes, as has been stated, research is done to determine the safety and/or efficacy of "nonvalidated practices." In such research the relationship between the physician-investigator and patient-subject is more complex than either a physician-patient or investigator-subject relationship. In order to determine whether it is justified to proceed with the total activity or with any of its component parts, it is necessary to analyze each of the component parts for what it really is. The employment of a maneuver that may be classified as a nonvalidated practice is not in and of itself research. As Mr. Chayet has pointed out, it may be malpractice—but it is not research. The fact that most of us have a tendency to define an activity as research merely because it entails a maneuver that is nonvalidated not only does not help us solve any problems—for example, whether employment of the maneuver is justified—but it also tends to give research a bad name.

Parenthetically, I must take exception to Mr. Chayet's suggestion that the earliest malpractice case—*Slater v. Baker and Stapleton* (6)—involved research. This was not an effort to develop generalizable knowledge; it did not even involve the use of a nonvalidated practice. It was a pointlessly destructive act about which Mr. Slater complained. The judge in the case called the wrongful act an experiment (according to a dictionary definition of the word, it was). Many of us, however, tend to use the words "experimentation" and "research" interchangeably. When we begin to discuss things of the sort Mr. Baker (the surgeon) did as research, we contribute to tarnishing the public image of research.

Nonvalidated practice has much more in common with validated practice than it has with research. The decision to use a nonvalidated diagnostic procedure or therapeutic modality should ordinarily be made in the same way that one makes the decision to use a validated procedure. That is, of the various modalities or procedures available to accomplish the purpose agreed upon by the physician and patient, this one seems most likely to achieve the shared objective and least likely to produce adverse effects. In this case, it makes sense to talk about alternatives as required in DHEW guidelines for informed consent. A choice between the various alternatives may be based on those factors that seem most important to the patient—e.g., risk, benefit, inconvenience, expense. In research there are no such alternatives from which to choose. The only alternatives are to do it or not to do it. The requirement for an explication of alternatives—derived from the medical practice model—clearly is inapplicable to research.

In the complex activity commonly called therapeutic research, the components that would properly be called research are those designed to establish the safety and/or efficacy of the nonvalidated practice. These are virtually never done for the benefit of the individual patient or subject. They are always designed to contribute to generalizable knowledge. While they can always be rejected without jeopardy to the life or health of the patient, the nonvalidated practice often cannot.

The Risks of Research

There is a widely held belief that assuming the role of research subject is a highly risky business. This assumption is clearly reflected in the legislative history of P.L. 93-348 (28); it is further reflected in the deliberations of the Commission that this act created. For example, because the Commission considered the role of research subject a hazardous occupation, it called upon a philosopher to analyze the distinctions between this and other hazardous occupations (37). But as some empirical data become available, the role of research subject does not seem to be particularly dangerous. Arnold (38, p. 18) has analyzed the risks of being a subject in Phase I drug testing—that most maligned of research activities. According to his estimates, the risk of physical or psychological harm from Phase I drug testing is slightly greater than that involved in being an office secretary, one-seventh that of window washers, and one-ninth that of miners. Subsequently, Cardon et al. (39) reported the results of their large-scale survey of investigators designed to determine the incidence of injuries to research subjects. They found that in "non-therapeutic research," the risk of being disabled either temporarily or permanently was substantially less than that of being similarly harmed in an accident. None of their nearly 100,000 subjects of "non-therapeutic research" died. The risks of being a subject in "therapeutic research" were substantially higher. However, the risk either of disability (temporary or permanent) or fatality was substantially less than the risk of similar unfortunate outcomes in other medical settings involving no research.

Bernard Barber and his colleagues (40, pp. 47-51) reported that in the biomedical research studies they examined, the risk-benefit ratios could be characterized as "less favorable" in 18 percent and "least favorable" in 8 percent. While this statement is probably a true reflection of the situation they observed, it is profoundly misleading. Unfortunately, it has had a major impact on the development of public policy (28, p. 18); it also has had an effect on the public conception of the nature of research.

Let us analyze briefly how we have contributed to the creation of this true, yet misleading, statement. It is often stated that assuming the role of subject in biomedical research nearly always entails the assumption of some risk of either physical or psychological harm or—at least—inconvenience (41). To many members of the public and to many analysts of research involving human subjects who are not themselves researchers, the word "risk" seems to carry the implication that there is a possibility of some dreadful consequence; this is made to seem even more terrifying when it is acknowledged that, in some cases, the very nature of this dreadful consequence cannot be anticipated. And yet, it is so much more common that when biomedical researchers discuss risk, they mean a possibility that there might be something like a bruise after a venipuncture.

Further, as we discuss potential benefits of research, we tend to be cautious to point out that: "Ordinarily, the study is being done not for the benefit of the subject but rather for purposes of deriving information which may in the future be of benefit to others" (41). When we prepare protocols for presentation to the IRB and consent forms for presentation to prospective subjects, we group together all risks—whether of physical or psychological harm or of inconvenience. We are very careful to prepare comprehensive lists of risks. By contrast, we tend to minimize the use of language that might seem to promise benefit, and we emphasize the fact that we are searching for generalizable knowledge (41).

If I wish to draw venous blood from patients with schizophrenia for purposes of assaying monoamine oxidase activity, it is quite possible to prepare a consent form that will not disturb any person having a legitimate concern (e.g., IRB member, patient, sociologist). I can make it clear that there is a risk—there might be momentary pain and, perhaps, a bruise. There is, of course, no possibility of benefit to the individual. However, there is a possibility of learning something about schizophrenics in general and that, in some way I cannot predict, this knowledge might be used to develop improved diagnostic or therapeutic techniques. A social scientist examining this protocol and consent form with a binary system of classification of risks and benefits will find that there is risk but no possibility of benefit to the subject and no assurance of benefit to society. Thus, this will be classified as one of the "least favorable" risk-benefit ratios and I will be branded a "permissive" investigator (40, pp. 7-8).

To forestall the creation of such problems, I suggest a change in the language we use to discuss the risks of research so as to more accurately reflect the realities of the situation and, further, to facilitate the development of a language that we might more easily share with individuals who are not biomedical researchers. I have proposed the following classification of research activities based on the nature of the risks (42).

1. *Research presenting mere inconvenience to the subjects:* Research presenting the subject with the necessity of bearing the burden of mere inconvenience is distinguished from that presenting the possibility of consequential injury (determined as a function of probability and magnitude). Research in this category employs techniques, modalities, and interventions that have been tested sufficiently to earn the classification of accepted or approved (for either research or practice purposes). It is characterized as presenting no greater risk of consequential injury to the subject than that inherent in a prospective subject's particular life situation. It is not appropriate to consider risks irrelevant to the design or purpose of the research; for example, it usually inappropriate to calculate the risks of being injured in an automobile accident (42, p. 8).

This class of research is by far the most common. In general, what we ask is that a prospective subject give of his or her time (to reside in a clinical research center, to be observed in a physiology laboratory, to fill out a questionnaire, to be interviewed, and so on). Often there is a request to draw some blood or to collect urine or feces.

2. *Research presenting known risk of physical or psychological harm:* Research in this category employs techniques, modalities, and interventions that have been tested sufficiently well to predict with reasonable certainty both the probability and magnitude of physical or psychological harm. In the case of prophylactic, diagnostic, or therapeutic maneuvers, they have been tested sufficiently well to be classified as accepted or approved. The probability and/or magnitude of physical or psychological harm is greater than that inherent in the subject's life situation (42, pp. 12-13).

3. *Research presenting unknown risk of physical or psychological harm:* In this category the technique, modality, or intervention has not been performed sufficiently often or well in humans to permit a reasonable assessment of the probability and magnitude of the harm it might produce. In this category, for example, we find Phase I drug-testing activities (42, pp. 11-12).

There are other categories of research; one class that presents combinations of known and unknown risk includes most of the research we do to test the safety and efficacy of nonvalidated practices. The concept of unknown risk of unknown harm may be particularly frightening to the public. Thus, it is essential to emphasize in our discussions of these categories of research that, while an honest expression of our state of knowledge forces us to acknowledge that things—even dreadful things—might happen, the nature of which we cannot predict, our experience is that they very rarely do (42, pp. 64-68).

In our discussions of risks, we have a penchant for focusing on those of physical or psychological harm. However, there are also economic, social, and legal risks presented by various kinds of biomedical research (43); these must be dealt with differently (42, pp. 10-11, 47-51). Additionally, in some kinds of research the major burdens of risk are borne not by the individual subjects, but rather by society, institutions, or classes of people (42, pp. 16-29).

We should proceed promptly to correct the language we use to describe the risks of research. Until we do, we can expect to see reiterations of the kinds of errors that we find in the studies of Barber et al. (40). In fact, the very same types of problems may be found in a recently completed large-scale survey of IRB function (44).

We should also make it very clear that most research—even that research commonly called nontherapeutic—presents the risk of inconvenience as distinguished from physical or psychological harm. If we do, we might begin to see more satisfactory analyses of the circumstances under which proxy consent is acceptable (35) and more felicitous criteria proposed for the selection of subjects (45).

Institutional Bureaucracy

Mr. Chayet has expressed grave concern with the increasing regulatory requirement for the establishment in research institutions of time- and energy-consuming yet questionably effective bureaucracy. His expressions of alarm about some of the things on which he has chosen to comment are excessive. On the other hand, he has not mentioned some of the most alarming new developments.

For example, Mr. Chayet states that "many of the presently constituted IRBs are illegal because they do not have the requisite number of community representatives." Since, according to present DHEW regulations, the requisite number is one, it is difficult to imagine that "there are simply not enough people available to serve on the committees that presently exist."

His discussion of the proposal for the establishment of Organizational Review Committees (ORCs) in the August 23, 1974 DHEW proposal (18) and his enumeration of the tasks assigned to them seems to imply that this is something new. In fact, the ORC is the IRB. As one follows the evolution of federal regulation describing committees to provide what was at first called "group consideration," one finds many names assigned to them; ORC is but one. Since the passage of P.L. 93-348 in which Congress assigned the generic name IRB to these committees, there has been a tendency to develop a more uniform language in discussing them. This should help. The tasks that Mr. Chayet mentions that would be assigned to the ORC (now named IRB) are the traditional tasks assigned to these committees; they represent nothing new. Therefore, again, his alarm seems excessive.

But the news is not all good. Diligent readers of the Federal Register can always find something that is really alarming. For example, the August 17, 1976 proposal by the Energy Research and Development Administration (ERDA) contains the following statement (46) on the composition of the IRB: "No board shall consist of a majority of persons who are officers, employees, or agents of, or are otherwise associated with the institution, apart from their membership on the board." If this statement appears in the final regulation, Mr. Chayet's concern that there might not be enough people to go around might become a reality. For another example, the August 20, 1976 FDA proposal on medical devices (47) would hold the IRC (this is the same as the IRB, but, apparently, the FDA has not yet accepted the generic term) accountable for the veracity and completeness of the sponsor's statements about the device.

I must agree with Mr. Chayet that the establishment of Consent Committees (CCs) (19) would be a disaster; my reasons for opposing this proposal are published (48-50). The Commission, in its deliberations on research involving several classes of persons covered in the August 1974 DHEW proposal, has not yet found it necessary to recommend the development of CCs. It did not recommend that they not be developed; however, after hearing some of the arguments for and against them, the Commission—in its reports on research on the fetus and research on prisoners— was silent on the matter. The final DHEW regulations on research on the fetus—which reflect the Commission's recommendations—do not mention CCs; it seems that DHEW has abandoned its proposal to establish them. I find this encouraging.

I do not know why Mr. Chayet finds it necessary to recommend the presence of a "patient surrogate" who would "be able to fulfill the oft-lacking communication between the researcher and the subject." It seems to me that the "patient surrogate" proposal presents nearly all of the same problems as the CC (48-50). Such proposals have been made by others. Barbara Katz and Kenneth Rosenberg provided a rather unusual proposal— unusual in that it attempted to estimate the costs of its implementation—to the Commission. They suggested that in an acute inpatient facility there should be at least one full-time "patient advocate" per 50-100 patients and that in an ambulatory setting there should be one advocate per 1-2 doctors. Since they were discussing the need for such persons in general medical settings, I assume that even larger numbers would be necessary in the institutional environments in which most neuropsychopharmacologic research is conducted. Implementation of this proposal would clearly cost a lot of money, time, and energy. Even more important to me is the fact that such proposals reflect an assumption of distrust within an institution, which—in my view—is enormously destructive (48, 50). Further, I have argued that the arbitrary superimposition of a third party on the consent negotiations and other interactions between investigator and subject will be contrary to the intent of the requirement for negotiating informed consent in the first place (49, p. 48). It is a potential invasion of privacy; in many cases, such a requirement is tantamount to a declaration to the prospective subject that his or her judgment (ability to comprehend, ability or freedom to make choices, and so on) is to be questioned. If a major purpose of negotiating informed consent is to foster the expression of the prospective subject's autonomy, the imposition of a third party—whether or not the propsective subject wishes one—is contrary to this purpose; it is paternalistic in the worst sense of the word. I therefore suggest that third parties should be made available if and when the subject wishes to have one. The subject should be allowed to choose the type of person who would be most suitable for the occasion. Only in extraordinary circumstances should there be a requirement for a third-party scrutinizer of the interactions between the investigator and subject (49, pp. 46-52). This requirement should be imposed by the IRB on a protocol-by-protocol basis. I would be most sad to see such a requirement created in federal regulation for a class of research activities; inevitably it would be overused to the detriment of all concerned.

Conclusions

There are some very serious conceptual and semantic problems that tend to undermine most of our efforts to discuss the law as it relates to research. Three of the more important are: (a) We fail to distinguish adequately between research, on one hand, and the accepted and routine practice of medicine, on the other. (b) We distinguish therapeutic from nontherapeutic research as if these were two distinct sets of activities and, further, as if the distinction—if it could be made—would be meaningful. (c) We tend incorrectly to view research as a highly risky business and the role of research subject as a hazardous occupation. This commentary illustrates some of the adverse consequences of these conceptual and semantic problems. We find discussions with each other difficult, and communications with the public and its representatives nearly impossible. We reach wrong conclusions in our ethical analyses and—based on them—develop inappropriate ethical norms, guidelines, and regulations. Our confusion contributes to the creation of a bad public image for research. Specific proposals are offered that should lead to the resolution of some of these problems.

While I agree with Mr. Chayet that it is simply impossible to regulate everything, I do not agree that the "intelligent dismantling of the bureaucracy" is a meaningful objective. Instead, I think that we should improve our bureaucracy and learn how to use it better. One important thing we could do is to hold the bureaucracy accountable only for the performance of meaningful functions. I agree that improved communication between the biomedical research community and public is essential. My approach to this would be to employ a language that could be understood by all participants. I disagree most strenuously with Mr. Chayet's proposal of a "patient surrogate" who might supply the deficiencies in communications between the researcher and the subject. Instead, in the usual case, I would offer the prospective subject the *option* of including a third party in his or her interactions with the investigator and, further, allow the subject to select the type of person most suitable. Only in unusual circumstances would I impose a requirement for a third-party scrutinizer of the interactions between the investigator and subject; these circumstances should be determined by the IRB on a protocol-by-protocol basis—not through regulation on a categorical basis.

MR. CHAYET: In order to correct a possible misinterpretation about my opinion regarding the presently constituted IRBs, I was referring to state regulations such as those in Massachusetts which have greatly increased the number of representatives required.

MS. HOLDER: My comments on Mr. Chayet's paper generally involve differences in emphasis, not basic disagreement with the thrust of his suggestions. He seems to believe that researchers are properly guardians of the rights of subjects. To disagree with such an assumption is not to question the good faith of the researchers; it is merely to indicate that the philosophical assumption of a democracy is that the legal system should facilitate each individual's ability to be the guardian of his own. The system is by no means perfect, but no system is any better than the people involved, and no matter how strict the regulations, their actual effectiveness is no better than the concern any researcher feels for his subject's rights. No IRB or patients' rights committee, no court, and no legislature can compensate for lack of concern for a patient or a subject; it is also probable that by the age at which one begins medical school, no educational institution can affect one's basic human values. However, what the requirements of all these groups can do and, I think, actually do is to increase awareness among researchers that human rights are involved and to enable them to fuse their pre-existing concerns with their knowledge. The result is compliance, quite willingly, with reasonable and sensible requirements.

The current problem, however, is that new regulations about a good idea, informed consent, are becoming so ludicrous, as Dr. Levine and I have pointed out about requirements for consent to research on tissue removed at surgery (51), that physicians are beginning to feel that consent and the philosophical concepts behind it are nothing but further manifestations of red tape. The essential aspects of the negotiating process are buried in trivia. As Prohibition and the current state of the marihuana laws demonstrate, when regulations of any sort do not appear sensible to the people whose behavior must conform to them, the inevitable result is a generalized contempt for the entire system of regulation, including its highly desirable aspects. This appears to me, as well as to Mr. Chayet, to be occurring today in the field of medical research, but that does not dissuade me from the view that research does require regulation beyond that imposed by the reseacher's own principles.

In turning to the specific subjects Mr. Chayet discusses, however, I disagree with his view that overregulation has actually occurred. There is a higher right in our society than the right to be free from disease and that is the right to be let alone (52). Even if treatment will improve or perhaps cure a patient, the right of a competent person to refuse it is quite clear. In one case, a schizophrenic who declined a mastectomy during a lucid interval was upheld in her right to do so in a subsequent court action (53), and other cases have involved the rights of elderly patients to refuse treatment for life-threatening illness (54, 55). No person has the right to condemn his child to die by refusing to allow treatment, but he most certainly has the right to refuse it for himself, regardless of the eccentricities of his personal risk-benefit analysis. Whatever benefits our society might derive from discovering how to cure diseases would be, in my opinion, much less important than the loss of the individual's right of choice that might be required in the process. I am puzzled by those who talk about "a right to health." If this concept is extended beyond a legal right of access to available facilities, questions arise as to what is a "right" (beyond that which a court is empowered to require of a party to a lawsuit) and what is "health." Beyond that, however, I would object to being compelled to be healthy. There may be a right; there certainly is no duty.

For this reason, I particularly dissent from Mr. Chayet's view that at least some nondangerous, mentally ill persons would be better off in institutions where they receive better physical care than wandering about untreated in hostile communities. I entirely agree with his concerns, and I would hope that mental health professionals and physicians of all types who deal with such persons would make strenuous efforts to persuade them to seek out, voluntarily, available therapy, and I would hope that the therapy would be of the highest possible level; but if no treatment is available or if they choose to decline it, freedom to sleep on a park bench instead of in an institution is itself a value I feel should be preserved. As a well-known song says, freedom may be "another word for nothing left to lose," but I am still prepared to defend it. Adequate provision of help and care to those who need it and want it is years away in this country, and I, for one, am prepared to argue the right to harmless eccentricity, even though it may offend the community's aesthetic sense to see these people in our midst. Furthermore, psychiatric treatment, more than any other, requires the cooperation of the patient, so the therapeutic effect of compulsory treatment may in fact be negligible (56). Until all the people who desperately want help are receiving it at an adequate level, attempts to treat those who don't want it would seem to be an extraordinary waste of resources.

I am not at all opposed in principle to the concept of involuntary commitment. There are people whose illnesses are dangerous. Whether it be a contagious disease or mental illness leading to violent behavior, and whether or not effective treatment is available, the community deserves protection from them. I am also aware, however, that a good number of heroes and heroines in world history were probably fortunate to have lived prior to the "invention" of psychiatry. I have in mind particularly Joan of Arc. She was obviously a most peculiar girl, by the standards of her time and ours, and today, any physician informed about her story of hearing voices would be tempted to put her in a hospital.

I also disagree with Mr. Chayet's generalizations from the *Kaimowitz* (4) opinion about the effects that case may have on research. While it may well have been, as Mr. Chayet states, "a deliberate attempt to halt all research with institutionalized mentally ill individuals," the case did not succeed in doing so. As Mr. Chayet and I will undoubtedly agree, cases are filed every day, particularly against physicians, for reasons that border on the ludicrous, and most of them are thrown out of court. The philosophical motivations of plaintiffs are largely irrelevant because what matters are the judges' opinions. Anyone can sue anyone else for practically anything; winning and establishing a precedent is another matter.

The *Kaimowitz* decision quite specifically restricted itself to intrusive, irreversible procedures on the brain and the opinion stated clearly: "Any experimentation on the human brain, especially when it involves an intrusive irreversible procedure in a non-life-threatening situation should be undertaken with extreme caution and then only when answers cannot be obtained from animal experimentation *and from non-intrusive human experimentation*" (4) (emphasis supplied). The court, in fact, specifically stated that "other avenues of research must be utilized and developed," which hardly indicates that the three judges felt it should be prohibited. The entire discussion of the consent issue involved many explicit and implicit references to the fact that the procedure was surgical. An analogy might be made to the current state of the law involving a minor girl's right to receive contraception without parental consent. With one exception, all the reported cases have held that a teenage girl's right to privacy allows her to give a valid consent to prescription for birth control pills, and that her constitutional rights have been violated if she is refused medical service for this purpose from a governmentally supported facility because she refuses to ask for parental consent (57-60). It is highly improbable, however, that any court would also rule that a teenage girl was capable of giving a valid consent to a tubal ligation, even if she insisted that she was quite sure that she would never want to have children, a statement that would probably be accepted at face value by an obstetrician if made by a woman of 35. The irreversibility of surgery in both situations makes them *sui generis,* and thus general principles simply cannot be derived from them which are applicable to other forms of research with the involuntarily confined or to contraception for minors.

The next point in my disagreement with Mr. Chayet is in regard to his view that some aspects of the current informed-consent law have made it virtually impossible to do research with incompetent patients and that this is unfortunate. This question is concerned with another aspect of freedom and the value we place on it. I would not personally object to a situation in which only those patients who had guardians who were family members could be used as research subjects if they themselves could not understand the consent negotiations. This procedure would at least eliminate such practices as occurred in the case at the Jewish Chronic Disease Hospital where senile patients were used as subjects. The litigation arising from that situation did not involve any of the subjects as parties. They never had anyone speak for them as individuals, even after the publicity given to the case (57). While obtaining consent from guardians is admittedly inconvenient, the alternative is no consent at all, and the inevitable result of that is secret research. Unless the community as a whole is willing to accept the notion of unrestricted research, then having it out in the open where people can observe it and know about it is the best defense against exploitation of the helpless that we can devise. Even if there is only one researcher in the country whose desire for recognition and academic tenure is stronger than his concern for the autonomy of his subjects, it seems to me that it is necessary to create moderate inconvenience for everyone else in order to prevent him from such exploitation.

But is the situation really as bad as all that? Presumably most of these patients, however disturbed, even delusional, communicate in some way to their therapists. There are of course many patients who are unable to communicate. However, with those patients who can communicate, the psychiatrist should be capable of explaining the research project and inviting the patient to participate; otherwise, there may be some question about his abilities as well as the patient's. As Mr. Chayet points out, hospitalization, even involuntary hospitalization, usually does not mean that the patient cannot give a valid consent in law. For those patients who are legally incompetent or who are actually incapable, the same guardian who controls the patient's estate and makes other decisions appears to be the proper person to decide. There may be truly incompetent patients without guardians, but the possibility of forbidding research with them does not disturb me as much as does the possibility of research with incompetents that no one knows about, for the very same reasons that courts have held for several hundred years that judicial proceedings cannot be kept secret. A simple requirement of openness in any activity can, in itself, prevent a variety of abuses.

Proxy consent in an individual case may in fact be insufficient to protect the patient's rights. For example, there has been a great deal of criticism from within the medical profession as well as without about the Willowbrook experiments on hepatitis, and no one has questioned the fact that parents gave signed consents for each child (35, pp. 47-54). Proxy consent, however, is probably the best that can be done and it certainly would seem dangerous to abolish it.

Mr. Chayet does not make clear the distinctions between consent to research and consent to therapy. There may be life-threatening consequences from an inability to obtain consent to therapy for an incompetent, but research is not in the same category. Since the researcher's primary intent is to seek knowledge, not to benefit the particular patient (although he may also hope the patient improves), it cannot be assumed, as it is in treatment, that the patient's best interest is the paramount goal. Therefore, it is particularly necessary to afford the greatest protection possible to that subject who is incapable of comprehension because he is the most helpless member of society.

No court has ever indicated that the doctrine of therapeutic privilege is no longer permissible in the context of treatment, but the principles underlying it are simply inappropriate in the context of research. Whatever a sick person should or should not be told, at minimum he must understand that whatever is customarily done for his condition is being varied in some way for him and that the researcher is not solely motivated by a desire to promote his best interests. Failure to disclose that a surgical procedure was experimental without proof that the subject's death was the result of negligence has been held sufficient to support an action for damages (61).

None of the proxy consent cases cited by Mr. Chayet involved research. They involved minor or adult-incompetent donors of skin (11) or kidneys (10, 12). In those cases where the permission of the court was denied, I hope it is realized that most reserach protocols do not involve procedures as risky as surgery to remove a kidney. Furthermore, in most cases, the guardian of an incompetent has already been appointed at the time of the finding of incompetency and in almost no case would it be necessary to appoint a guardian solely for the purpose of consenting to proposed research. Any committed person whose estate is sufficiently substantial to require, for example, an inventory, as Mr. Chayet mentions, has assuredly had a guardian appointed at the time of hospitalization to administer financial affairs. If, as Mr. Chayet believes, guardians, in general, refuse to consent to research, it might be that they have legitimate objections to whatever project has been suggested to them since anything that could be of substantial benefit to their ward would presumably be welcomed.

I thoroughly agree with Mr. Chayet's position that good public relations between researcher and community will materially improve the environment in which research is conducted in this country. I would, however, suggest that openness about research and strict attention to the rights of subjects are probably more effective public relations moves than self-serving political action.

DR. MAY: I was really very glad to hear Ms. Holder say that researchers have rights too. It has troubled me that we always hear about the rights of society and, really, it seems to me that society is composed of a whole lot of different groups of individuals and you can classify those individuals one way or another, and all these groups have rights. They have duties and responsibilities, too, and there will always be a relative balance between responsibility to society and individual rights.

Mr. Chayet said that we need to get the attention of some of these bureaucracies and to support them. While I feel that perhaps we need to get their attention, I'm not prepared to support what some of these bureaucracies do. At one time I was working simultaneously for three bureaucracies, and none of them had a code of ethics for bureaucrats. We have developed a code of ethics for research investigators—and we worked on this task in a very earnest manner; I think it is about time for someone to develop a code of ethics for bureaucrats. I have seen many times when bureaucrats dealt with situations in ways that, frankly, if I looked at them with a moralistic eye, really troubled me. I might not go so far as to say that they were outright liars or that they were deliberately deceitful in their behavior, but certainly the truth was spun in ways that I do not feel that it should be spun. And there are ways of concealing information that I feel are not entirely ethical. I think it is just about time that we stimulate the bureaucrats to develop some overt codes of ethical behavior.

I wouldn't in any way presume to be an authority on legal problems, but there has been one type of problem that has considerably interested me. On one occasion, I suggested that our research bureaucratic agencies and our regulatory agencies had a duty to see that a patient who was given a drug that produced a therapeutic response would be continued on that research medication. I stated that they had an ethical responsibility to see that that particular patient should be entitled to continue on that drug if it had benefited him; and the shocked silence that this opinion generated was appalling. Really, I almost thought I was going to be drummed out of the society for making an improper suggestion. I think that we do need to pay more attention to such problems.

DR. GREENBLATT: I was delighted to hear the legal minds at work. My own experience has been that in order to survive in a bureaucracy you need legal help. When I was Commissioner in Massachusetts, we had several lawyers around; thus, I stayed out of jail. When I was Superintendent of Boston State Hospital, I had Neil Chayet around to help me consider the rights of patients. He was one of the first lawyers to study systematically patients living in the hospital in order to tell us what rights were being neglected. I remember so well when he came to my office after being on the wards for some time and said, "You have got an absolute, infinite number of needs, legal needs, for your patients," and we worried together how they would ever be satisfied.

While we have the legal minds here, I have been struggling to try to figure out what are the rights of patients. For example, does a patient have a right to treatment? I thought that was true when the *Rouse* case (62) was adjudicated, but that seems to be valid only for the District of Columbia.

Other cases that have come before higher courts, it seems to me, have emphasized the right to be free, but not the right to receive treatment. In the recent case of *Donaldson v. O'Connor* (3), the essential phrase was that "you cannot hold a patient who is nondangerous without more." The court didn't say what the "more" was, but you just can't hold them.

So it seems to me that all the discussions about the right to treatment come down to defining further the rights of the patient to be free to choose his place of abode, and dangerousness would be the primary criterion for holding the patient and no more. It seems to me that the higher courts have been reluctant to declare that all Americans have a right to treatment. There is a lot of sense to this reluctance because, frankly, we don't have the resources to treat all the patients.

I was just wondering if we could take advantage of the legal talent we have assembled to clarify that point.

Mr. Chayet raised the issue of politicization of professionals and professional organizations, and it is true that we are being progressively politicized. As I look back on the years, court decisions have progressively intruded on the right to treat. The right to treat now has to be redefined. I think that no vigorous professional societies are unpoliticized today. I therefore suggest that this organization, in which I have a real personal stake, start to think more in terms of the interface between it and the political area, and do let the press in. However, if we are going to let the press in and if we are going to be giving information to the press, that should not be done willy-nilly. I do not think that merely by possession of an M.D. degree we are thereby experts in public relations. We probably ought to have somebody schooled in public relations to assist with this interface to get the most out of it.

The other suggestion which appeals to me—although I don't know how we would implement it—is that every professional organization ought to have one or more citizen arms associated with it—citizen groups that you could turn to and who would have much more impact on legislators and the public than the organization itself, because the organization is always suspect for its personal interests.

MR. SCOTT: I was very happy to hear Angela Holder say something in defense of the *Kaimowitz* (4) case. I notice that a large number of participants have been very critical of the *Kaimowitz* decision. I would like to make one or two points about that decision to cast it in a more favorable light.

Some of the presenters and discussants have indicated that the *Kaimowitz* case means that mentally ill or persons who are prisoners cannot give consent to experimental treatment. Actually, the *Kaimowtiz* case says something much less than that. The *Kaimowitz* case involved an individual who had been confined indeterminately, that is, for the rest of his life, until such time as he was able to satisfy courts that he was psychologically fit and safe to be back in the community. The court in that situation said when a person has that much at stake in improving his mental condition, that person cannot voluntarily and competently give consent to so hazardous a procedure, as psychosurgery was known to be at that point.

I think the real flaw, if there was one in the *Kaimowitz* situation, was not with the court's determination. The flaw in that case was our approach toward people we consider to be dangerous, particularly those we consider to be sexually dangerous—that our legal system allows an individual to be put away for the rest of his life until such time as he can produce evidence that he is psychologically safe for release to the community.

DR. GALLANT: Mr. Chayet has reviewed the DHEW and FDA regulatory guidelines for human research as well as some litigation concerned with patient rights to treatment. It must be emphasized, however, that the regulations reviewed do *not* consider those research endeavors conducted by investigators not affiliated with institutions and not utilizing federal funds (63). At present, it is in this particular area of research that unethical conduct is more likely to occur. It is quite obvious that the federal regulations will have to be revised to cover all areas of research, federally funded or not.

Hopefully, the NCPHSBBR, which was established by Congress in 1974 as an advisory body to DHEW, will be replaced by a long-term National Advisory Council that will deal with the issues relating to federally and nonfederally funded research. Government regulations are aimed chiefly at federally funded programs; all persons serving as subjects in other research require similar protection. Hopefully, the Commission will also offer guidelines for the review committees, and some suggestions have been made that a hierarchy of such committees be composed of scientists, lawyers, theologians, and representatives of the human research population under investigation. A regional appeal board composed of similar types of representatives should exist for those situations in which the decisions of the local board are considered unsatisfactory. At the top of this hierarchy, a National Human Review Board should be established with a composition similar to that of the local boards, and this national board should also have the authority to evolve review standards and clarify questions of research and informed consent as they arise.

Concerning research with prisoners, some investigators believe that the guidelines for membership of the Protection Committees for Prisoner Research have not been wisely thought out in the regulations (64). There is an underlying assumption in these regulations that professional staffs of institutions would be less concerned about the patients' welfare than would lay members associated with the study. As part of my experience in research, I have attended meetings of IRBs composed of lay members as well as of researchers, clergymen, etc. The laymen, unless very carefully selected, frequently appear to be the most bored, and, as would be expected, the more complicated the research proposal, the more bored are the laymen. The restriction that no more than one-third of the members on the Protection Committee for Prison Research shall be scientists engaged in biomedical research or physicians will in all probability result in a lessening of the competence of the Protection Committee.

Research with children does provide additional ethical and legal problems and should receive additional attention. I would like to refer to the FDA report on guidelines for testing drugs in children (65). The two principal recommendations in this report were: (a) studies should be conducted with children only after the test drugs have been shown to be reasonably safe and effective in adults; and (b) tests should be conducted only with those children who need treatment and who stand to benefit directly from the studies in which they are involved. The latter recommendation is contrary to the decision in the *Bonner v. Moran* case (11), which Mr. Chayet cited, and thus researchers of childhood diseases are still in a quandary in regard to their legal status.

Unfortunately, in some specific disorders unique to children, such as childhood autism, prior demonstration of drug efficacy in adults may be irrelevant. In the use of methylphenidate, an efficacious and relatively safe drug for hyperkinetic children with minimal brain dysfunction, prior studies in adults would have been inappropriate, particularly since the drug has a potential for abuse and addiction in adults. These recommendations to the FDA did not show sufficient forethought, despite the fact that the Advisory Scientific Committee was composed of a number of outstanding pediatricians. Thus, excepting unusual emergency situations, it is essential to disseminate such reports widely at least six to twelve months in advance of publication in the Federal Register. Regulations concerning pediatric informed consent are desirable, but the problem cited above, as well as the recommended need to obtain consent from patients seven years of age or older, create unnecessary problems. In regard to the consent mechanism in children, if this mechanism is employed too early, the relative lack of comprehension will make consent meaningless. In fact, it is my very strong opinion that with patients who have limited capacity to consent, unless it is clear that the common-sense doctrine that those closest to the patient will best guard his interest has failed, the burden of proof is on those who will delegate such responsibilities to legal counsel or the court. However, I do agree with Mr. Chayet's recommendation about the use of a third party to aid the communication between the researcher and the subject. The use of the term "patient surrogate" is much more appropriate than the term "patient advocate" which immediately connotes a defense by argument. "Surrogate," which infers a representative or deputy of the patient, would be a more suitable title for the person aiding the informed-consent procedure in especially vulnerable patient populations. The "surrogate" is not proposed as an alternative to a Human Research Committee or an IRB, but rather as an addition to the review procedures. Surrogate or advocate consent is not recommended for the mentally competent patient who is not exposed to unusual external pressures. I do agree with Dr. Levine's statement that the requirement of a patient surrogate should be imposed by the IRB on a protocol-by-protocol basis, not by federal regulations "for a class of research activities."

I have to disagree with Ms. Holder's generalization that "the researcher's primary intent is to seek knowledge, not to benefit the particular patient . . . ." This is not always the case in psychopharmacologic research with severely ill, chronic schizophrenic patients. In this population, we usually select "drug-refractory" patients in order to expose them to the potential therapeutic benefits of a new agent. If therapeutic intent was not the primary goal, a random sampling of these patients, rather than a selection of "drug-refractory" subjects, would be more desirable from a methodological viewpoint.

In regard to the effect of recent regulations on drug development and the practice of medicine, there have been few competent comparisons between the United States and other countries. The only detailed comparative analysis showed that Britain, with less restrictive regulations, produced nearly four times as many new (single chemical entity) drugs as the United States during the years 1962-1971 (66). When examined by therapeutic category, the drug lags were most notable in the cardiovascular, gastrointestinal, diuretic, and antibacterial therapies. According to Wardell (66), the British place more reliance on evaluation and regulation, and there is better postmarketing drug surveillance in Britain. In this study, the lack of American awareness of the new drugs was even more surprising. In summary, Wardell believes that clearly discernible gains were made in Britain by introducing useful new drugs either earlier or more rapidly than in the United States. Another conclusion by Wardell was that recognized medical centers and teaching hospitals in the United States should be allowed to use investigational drugs for therapy at their own discretion as in Sweden and to do careful surveillance of these new drugs to obtain additional information while they are helping their patients. While the low number of new drugs in some categories in the United States may indicate industrial efforts to concentrate research on more effective drugs, recent events with the FDA, such as reaction of several very promising neuroleptic agents on the basis of mice carcinogenic studies, without outside expert consultation prior to the decision, forebode even more overly restrictive approaches which may effectively eliminate future efforts of pharmaceutical firms and research psychopharmacologists in this area. It appears that the decisions of governmental personnel, many of whom lack the necessary basic scientific and/or clinical expertise in the fields they are judging, may be more detrimental to the progress of psychopharmacology than recent new regulations or litigation. One of the drugs was an effective antischizophrenic agent which had the theoretical potential of producing minimal or no symptoms of tardive dyskinesia, a disabling, long-term neurologic side effect noted with almost all of the presently available neuroleptic agents for schizophrenia.

MR. FORCE: The suggested use of "patient surrogates" is tempting. However, before we commit ourselves to such an innovation, two areas must be clarified. The first has already been alluded to, that is, in which situations would it be appropriate to use a patient surrogate? The second question may be asked with regard to both the "patient surrogate" and the "patient advocate." What role should the lawyer play in decision making? In advancing the interests of his client or charge, shouldn't the surrogate or advocate be guided by fixed standards that are uniformly applicable? There might be a difference in the manner in which the lawyer fulfills his responsibilities depending on whether he is attempting to view the situation in terms of: (a) what he thinks is best for the patient or subject; (b) what he thinks the patient or subject would do if he were competent; (c) what he would do if he were in the patient or subject's position; or (d) what he thinks the ordinary person would do if he were in the patient or subject's position.

Despite some recent improvements, we know that overall the role of lawyers in "protecting" the interests of their clients in commitment proceedings has not been impressive (67). Therefore, until lawyers or others selected to perform the surrogate function have acquired adequate scientific expertise, they, like judges, must insist on scrupulous adherence to required legal procedures such as approval by the requisite IRB, compliance with informed-consent prerequisites, investigation of possible conflicts of interest, and objection to research or treatment that "shocks the conscience."

One other reservation I have is that, after time, the surrogate might perform his duties routinely and be co-opted by the "system." The presence of the surrogate, like the giving of *Miranda* (68) warnings, might serve to insulate rather than dispel overreaching.

REFERENCES

1. U.S. Senate, Committee on the Judiciary, Subcommittee on Constitutional Rights. *Individual Rights and the Federal Role in Behavior Modification.* Washington, D.C.: 1974.
2. *Wyatt v. Stickney,* 344 F. Supp. 387 (M.D. Ala. 1972).
3. *Donaldson v. O'Connor,* 422 U.S. 563 (1975).
4. *Kaimowitz v. Department of Mental Health of the State of Michigan,* Civ. Op. No. 73-19434 AW (Cir Ct. Wayne County, Mich., 1973). This decision was not published officially but may be found in two casebooks: Miller, W., Dawson, R.O., Dix, G.E., and Parnas, R.I. *The Mental Health Process,* 2nd ed. Mineola, N.Y.: New York Foundation Press, 1976, p. 567 and Brooks, A.D. *Law Psychiatry and the Mental Health System.* Boston: Little, Brown, 1974, p. 902.
5. *Jobes et al. v. Michigan Department of Mental Health et al.,* File No. 74 004 130 D.C.
6. *Slater v. Baker and Stapleton,* C.B., 95 Eng. Rep. 860 (1767).
7. *Mohr v. Williams,* 95 Minn. 261 (1904).
8. *Dunham v. Wright,* 423 F. 2d 940, 941-942 (3rd Cir. 1970).
9. Declaration of Helsinki. *World Med. J.,* 11:281, 1964. Revised by the 29th World Medical Assembly, Tokyo, Japan, 1975.
10. *Strunk v. Strunk,* 445 S.W. 2d 145 (Ky. 1969).
11. *Bonner v. Moran,* 126 F. 2d 121 (D.C. Cir. 1941).
12. *In re Richardson,* 284 So. 2d 185 (La. App. 1973).
13. Neil Chayet: personal communication.
14. Mass. Gen. Laws, c. 272, sec. 71 (1931).
15. M.G.L.A., c. 112, sec. 12 J.
16. M.G.L.A., c. 94C, sec. 8 (i).
17. 45 CIT, Part 46.
18. 39 Fed. Reg. 30648 (Aug. 23, 1974).
19. 39 Fed. Reg. 30656, sec. 46.506 (a) (2) (Aug. 23, 1974).
20. Food, Drug and Cosmetic Act, 21 U.S.C.A., sec. 355 (e).

21. Food, Drug and Cosmetic Act, 21 U.S.C.A., sec. 355 (i).
22. 21 CFR, sec. 312.1.
23. National Research Act, P.L. 93-348, 42 U.S.C.A., sec. 289 1 (1974).
24. 45 CFR, sec. 46.3 (h).
25. *Clay v. Martin*, 509 F. 2d 109 (2nd Cir. 1975).
26. 39 Fed. Reg. 30655, sec. 46.503 (Aug. 23, 1974).
27. 39 Fed. Reg. 30655, sec. 46.501 (b).
28. Kay, E.M. Legislative history of Title II-Protection of human subjects of biomedical and behavioral research—of the National Research Act: P.L. 93-348. Prepared for the National Commission for the Protection of Human Subjects of Biomedical and Behavioral Research (NCPHSBBR), 1975.
29. Blumgart, H.L. In: *Experimentation with Human Subjects.* P.A. Freund, ed. New York: George Braziller, 1970, pp. 39-65.
30. Moore, F.D. In: *Experimentation with Human Subjects.* P.A. Freund, ed. New York: George Braziller, 1970, pp. 358-378.
31. Levine, R.J. The boundaries between biomedical or behavioral research and the accepted and routine practice of medicine. Prepared for the NCPHSBBR, 1975.
32. Levine, R.J. In: *Human Experimentation.* R.L. Bogomolny, ed. Dallas: SMU Press, 1976, pp. 3-20.
33. Levine, R.J. On the relevance of ethical principles and guidelines developed for research to health services conducted or supported by the Secretary, DHEW. Prepared for the NCPHSBBR, 1976.
34. Nuremberg Code (Judgement on Experimentation without Restriction). *United States v. Karl Brandt*, 1947. In: Katz, J. *Experimentation with Human Beings.* New York: Russel Sage Foundation, 1972, pp. 305-306.
35. Ramsey, P. *The Patient as Person.* New Haven: Yale University Press, 1970.
36. Fried, C. *Medical Experimentation: Personal Integrity and Social Policy.* New York: American Elsevier Publishing Co., 1974.
37. Wartofsky, M. On doing it for money. Prepared for the NCPHSBBR, 1976.
38. Arnold, J.D. Alternatives to the use of prisoners in research in the United States. Prepared for the NCPHSBBR, 1976.
39. Cardon, P.V., Dommel, F.W., Jr., and Trumble, R.R. *New Eng. J. Med.,* 295:650-654, 1976.
40. Barber, B., Lally, J.J., Makarushka, J.L., and Sullivan, D. *Research on Human Subjects.* New York: Russell Sage Foundation, 1973.
41. Levine, R.J. *Clin. Res.,* 22:42-46, 1974.
42. Levine, R.J. Appropriate guidelines for the selection of human subjects for participation in biomedical and behavioral research. Prepared for the NCPHSBBR, 1976.
43. Levine, R.J. *Bioethics Digest,* 1 (3):1-17, 1976.
44. Survey Research Center, Institute for Social Research, The University of Michigan. Research involving human subjects. Prepared for the NCPHSBBR, 1976.
45. Jonas, H. Philosophical reflections on experimenting with human subjects. In: *Experimentation with Human Subjects.* P.A. Freund, ed. New York: George Braziller, 1970, pp. 1-31.
46. Energy, Research, and Development Administration: Protection of human subjects: Proposed regulations. Federal Register 41 (No. 160): 34778-34782. August 17, 1976. Legal citation: 10 CFR 705.
47. Department of Health, Education, and Welfare—Food and Drug Administration: Medical devices: Proposed investigational device exemption. Federal Register 41 (No. 163): 35282-35313. August 20, 1976. Legal citation: 21 CFR 4, 6, 801.

48. American Federation for Clinical Research. *Clin. Res.*, 23:53-60, 1975.
49. Levine, R.J. The nature and definition of informed consent in various research settings. Prepared for the NCPHSBBR, 1975.
50. Levine, R.J. The institutional review board. Prepared for the NCPHSBBR, 1976.
51. Holder, A., and Levine, R.J. Informed consent for research on specimens obtained at autopsy or surgery: A case study in the overprotection of human subjects. *Clin. Res.*, 24:68, 1976.
52. *Olmstead v. United States,* 277 US 438 (1928) (Brandeis in dissent).
53. *In re Maida Yetter,* 62 Pa. D & C 2d 619 (Pa. 1973).
54. *In re Nemser,* 273 N.Y.S. 2d 624 (N.Y. 1966).
55. *Palm Springs General Hospital v. Martinez* (Fla. Cir. Ct., Dade County, 1971).
56. Katz, J. The right to treatment: An enchanting legal fiction? *U. Chicago Law Rev.*, 36:755, 1969.
57. Katz, J. *Experimentation with Human Beings.* New York: Russell Sage Foundation, 1972, Chapter I.
58. *T.H. v. Jones,* DC Utah (unpublished), cert. denied 48 L Ed 2d 811 (1976).
59. *Note:* Parental consent requirements and privacy rights of minors: The contraceptive controversy. *Harvard Law Rev.*, 88:1018, 1975.
60. *Population Services v. Wilson,* 398 F. Supp. 321 (DC N.Y. 1975).
61. *Fiorentino v. Wenger,* 227 NE 2d 296 (N.Y. 1967).
62. *Rouse v. Cameron,* 373 F. 2d 451 (D.C. 1966).
63. *The Institutional Guide to DHEW Policy on Protection of Human Subjects.* DHEW Pub. No. 72-102, Dec. 1, 1971.
64. Federal Register—DHEW—PHS. Protection of human subjects: Policies and procedures. Vol. 38 (No. 221):31743, Nov. 16, 1973.
65. FDA report: Guidelines for testing drugs in children. A report of the committee on drugs of the American Academy of Pediatrics to the FDA, DHEW, July, 1974.
66. Wardell, W.M. Drug development, regulation, and the practice of medicine. *JAMA*, 229:1457-1461, 1974.
67. Cohen, F. The function of the attorney and the commitment of the mentally ill. *Tex. Law Rev.*, 44:424-469, 1965-66.
68. *Miranda v. Arizona,* 384 U.S. 436 (1966).

CHAPTER IV

Ethical Issues in Psychopharmacologic Research

KAREN A. LEBACQZ

The range of ethical issues raised by neuropsychopharmacologic research is immense,[1] and the history of treatment of these issues is meager. I propose to raise three general questions about research ethics and six questions particularly pertinent to neuropsychopharmacologic research.

In general: (a) What justifications can be offered for the research enterprise? (b) How should subjects be selected, and is it justifiable to use patients in state mental hospitals? and (c) What are the requirements for "informed consent" to participate in research, and do those requirements preclude participation by institutionalized mental patients?

In particular: (a) Is incomplete disclosure of research design or risks justifiable? (b) Can research be conducted ethically when subjects are not able to withdraw at any time? (c) Is it ethical to induce a psychotomimetic state? (d) Can one morally give consent to change the consenting organ itself? (e) Can research inducing addiction be conducted ethically? and (f) What criteria should be used to measure "success" in neuropsychopharmacologic research?

---

[1] Since neuropsychopharmacologic research is done on children, dying people, prisoners, addicts, and others, it raises all the ethical dilemmas of research on the vulnerable, uncomprehending, or disadvantaged. To deal with all these issues is beyond the scope of this essay; the institutionalized mental patient will be discussed as a paradigmatic case.

I cannot provide answers to all these questions. Nor can I review and critique the various professional codes and governmental regulations under which neuropsychopharmacologic research is conducted.[2] I shall focus on the principles and modes of reasoning that provide a framework for analyzing ethical dilemmas in neuropsychopharmacologic research and on the need for future analysis in critical areas.

THE JUSTIFICATION FOR RESEARCH

Although medical research is widely accepted today as an integral part of health care delivery, demands for the protection of human research subjects occasionally threaten the research enterprise. For example, a 1973 Massachusetts law provided that "no person shall administer psychotropic drugs to [a pupil in any public school in the state] for the purposes of clinical research" (1). I would like to begin, therefore, by presenting several grounds on which the research enterprise can be justified.

Research is commonly justified by pointing to the benefits it produces. Research is an activity designed to contribute to generalizable knowledge (2), and knowledge itself may be seen as a good. In a "pill-taking culture" such as ours, simply learning about the effects of "mind-altering" drugs may be an important form of Socratic self-knowledge, and neuropsychopharmacologic research can be jusitifed because it brings us this knowledge (3, 4).

More often, it is not knowledge alone, but the medical and social benefits derived from that knowledge that are used to justify research. The development of specific drug interventions for schizophrenia and depression with a resulting shift away from hospitalization, for example, present justifications for neuropsychopharmacologic research (5-7).

Important though these benefits may be, there are problems in justifying research solely in terms of the benefits it produces. Not everyone agrees on what constitutes a "benefit." Opponents of the administration of ritalin to hyperactive children charge that quieting children down is not a "benefit" since it diverts attention from the need for better classroom environments. Indeed, some charge that any "chemical management" of people is a harm rather than a benefit (1). In a pluralistic society, what is a "benefit" to some is not to others.

---

[2] The proliferation of codes and regulations in the last ten years has led to an unfortunate identification of regulation with ethics. In the literature on neuropsychopharmacologic research, discussions of the "ethics" of research often take the form of criticism of current regulations. Since codes and regulations are intended, in part, to embody ethical principles by concretizing them for particular situations, this confusion is understandable. The question of how to implement ethical principles in regulation is an important one, but one which I cannot discuss here.

Even when advocates agree about the "benefits" to be produced, they may disagree about how those benefits are to be obtained. While agreeing that dying patients should be enabled to achieve a level of self-acceptance, some would argue for the use of LSD to that end, while others would advocate only psychotherapy and nonpharmacologic approaches. Our society accepts the use of pharmacologic agents for certain purposes (e.g., to foster pleasant conversation at parties), but not necessarily for others (e.g., to quiet restless children).

But suppose that we agree on the desirability of a certain end *and* on the acceptability of pharmacologic agents to reach that end. There are still problems in justifying neuropsychopharmacologic research solely in terms of the benefits it produces. It is not always possible to measure the benefits of an individual research project. Rarely does a single project bring about large social benefits. Rather, a project tests a hypothesis; completion of the project may narrow the field of hypotheses to be tested, but does not necessarily result in immediate improvements in patient management. It is always difficult to say, then, that the benefits of a particular piece of research will outweigh the possible risks involved. The benefits from research are cumulative, and more appropriately belong to the research enterprise as a totality.[3]

It therefore seems to me a mistake to look to the benefits produced as the sole justification for research. I propose two additional arguments.

First, some researchers complain that regulation of research has become so cumbersome that it stifles creativity. Similarly, others complain that regulation obstructs academic freedom. Implicit in such complaints is an assumption that curiosity, creativity, and freedom are human values to be fostered and that research is good in itself as an expression of these human values. Research is justified, therefore, not only by the goods it produces, but also by its intrinsic nature.[4] To the extent that respect for the autonomy of persons is a necessary condition of human society, expressions of autonomy, freedom, human creativity, and the like are to be respected regardless of the benefits they produce.

Second, research not only produces benefits, it prevents harms. Some medical interventions come to be accepted as routine practice without having been validated by careful research. Some of these interventions harm rather than help patients. Research is necessary to test the safety and efficacy of "routine" and "accepted" practices, so that harmful practices can be stopped. Since most people consider the moral imperative "do not harm" *(primum*

---

[3] For this reason, I am always skeptical of the requirement to assess the "risks and benefits" of a particular project and to declare that the "benefits" outweigh the "risks."

[4] These justifications are roughly analogous to the philosophical distinction between utilitarian and deontological modes of reasoning.

non nocere) to be more stringent than the imperative to do good, the recognition that research prevents harm provides a particularly compelling justification for the research enterprise.

SELECTION OF SUBJECTS

If we are to do research, on whom shall we do it? Is it permissible to use subjects who are "administratively convenient"? In trials of a new drug, is it preferable to use sick or healthy subjects? When, if ever, is it permissible to use children, prisoners, mentally retarded persons, or other vulnerable or noncomprehending people?

In a celebrated article, Hans Jonas (8) proposes that the ideal subjects for any research are those maximally able to identify with the goals of the research and understand its risks—namely, researchers themselves! The less one understands the risks of research and identifies with its purposes, the less permissible is it for one to be used as a subject in research. He thus establishes a "descending order of permissibility" in which those who are vulnerable, noncomprehending, sick, or "administratively convenient" would be used only when the pool of researchers and scientists had been diminished. By this criterion, it would occasionally be permissible to use vulnerable, institutionalized, or noncomprehending subjects, but it would never be *preferable* to use them.

Jonas derives his "descending order of permissibility" from the fundamental duty to respect persons by treating them as ends and not merely as means. The use of a person as a means to an end, as in research, is justified only if the person so identifies with the purposes of the research that participation in it becomes a genuine expression of his or her own will. In order for this to occur, the person must truly understand the purposes and risks of the research. Hence, researchers become the ideal subjects.

This system is clearly intended to protect those who are vulnerable and unable to protect themselves. While it has much initial appeal, it does present some problems.

First, researchers may not have the physiologic or psychologic characteristics needed to test the research hypothesis. As Levine (9) suggests, the first criterion for selection of a subject pool is that the potential subjects have the attributes that permit testing of the research hypothesis. If the hypothesis relates to the effects of a psychotropic drug on a particular mood state, the subjects must demonstrate that mood state. (Of course, if the research calls for "controls," researchers and other members of the scientific community *might* qualify as control subjects.) Objections have been raised to the use of healthy volunteers in Phase I drug testing because their physiology may so differ from that of the sick as to prevent any extrapolation of data from one group to the other; thus, the use of healthy volunteers may not permit testing of hypotheses relevant to the development of medical interventions. Contrary to Jonas's proposal that subjects be selected first from the pool of physicians and researchers, we might propose instead that subjects be selected first from those who are biologically or psychologically qualified in terms of the research design.

Moreover, one may question whether a system such as that proposed by Jonas might unjustly deprive some persons of benefits available to others. Participation in research is not always a "burden" (or "sacrifice," as Jonas calls it). The risks in most research are small, and the subjects may derive considerable benefit—financial or psychological—from participation. To the extent that participation is a benefit, a system would not be just if it unfairly prevented some persons from the opportunity to derive that benefit. In his concern to ensure a just distribution of the *burdens* of research, Jonas seems to ignore the distribution of *benefits*.

But suppose that there are several subject populations that could be used to test a hypothesis, and that among those subject populations some are more convenient to use—specifically, patients in state mental institutions. Is it just to use this population?

Clearly, the answer depends on how "justice" (or "injustice") is defined. I propose to review very briefly three alternative concepts of justice and their implications for the selection of subjects for research.

In one classical formulation (the utilitarian one), justice consists in maximizing goods for the community at large: "the greatest good for the greatest number." So long as "the greatest number" gain "the greatest good," state mental hospital patients or other vulnerable or uncomprehending persons could be used as subjects in research.[5] The criterion for selection of research subjects would be maximizing benefit and minimizing cost to society at large. There is no requirement that those who bear burdens should also reap benefits, nor is there special protection for the weak in this system.

A contrasting formulation of justice is the Marxist dictum: "From each according to his or her ability, to each according to his or her need." This dictum intends to protect the weak and require sacrifice from the strong. To the extent that participation in research is a burden, those who have least "ability" and greatest "need" ought not to be used as research subjects, but

---

[5] However, much depends on what is considered "good." If the use of vulnerable or noncomprehending subjects is considered dehumanizing, then it might be judged sufficiently evil to outweigh the good results of the research. A full utilitarian theory of justice requires a theory of the good.

should derive benefits from the research enterprise. Conversely, to the extent that participation in research is a benefit, it is precisely those who have least "ability" and most "need" who ought to be used as subjects so that they can reap the benefits of participation.

Recently, John Rawls has proposed yet a third formulation of the requirements of justice (10). For an institution or a system of distribution to be just, it must work to the advantage of the "least advantaged." While this theory sounds similar to the Marxist dictum, it has one very significant difference: anyone may bear burdens (not simply the powerful or able), so long as the system works to the advantage of the "least advantaged." In contrast to the utilitarian formula, it is not "the greatest number" who must benefit from the system, but rather the "disadvantaged."

Such a system does not exclude anyone *a priori* from being a research subject. Thus, it is not necessarily wrong to use state mental hospital patients as research subjects. Assuming that they are among the "least advantaged," however, it would be wrong to use them if they are thereby burdened and reap none of the benefits. For example, if most research involving risk is done in state mental institutions while the benefits arising from research go primarily to private patients and those who are more advantaged, then the system is unjust. (Our current system merits much scrutiny in this regard.) However, it is not wrong to use state mental hospital patients if such use redounds to their benefit.

The effectuation in social policy of any theory of justice is very complex. Consider, for example, the case of drug testing. Numerous advocates propose that drugs should be tested first in patients rather than in normal volunteers, so that those who bear the burdens of research will also reap the benefits. At first glance, such a concurrence between bearing burdens and reaping benefits would seem to ensure a kind of fundamental justice. But if patients are more "disadvantaged" than normal subjects (both because of their infirmities and because of their dependence on doctors or institutions), then the use of normal volunteers in a system designed to benefit the sick may be more just than the use of the patients themselves. By the same reasoning, the use of some normal populations would be more justifiable than the use of others.

Ethical issues regarding selection of subjects for research cannot be decided only in terms of the choice of subjects for each research protocol. It is the *system* of recruitment of volunteers for research, the distribution of the benefits and burdens of participation in research, and the distribution of the benefits accruing from the research enterprise that must be scrutinized. Much more work is needed on the justice of selection of subjects for research.

"INFORMED CONSENT" AND THE
INSTITUTIONALIZED MENTAL PATIENT

Following the atrocities of medical experimentation in Nazi Germany, the Nuremberg Code (11) and every subsequent major code governing research on human subjects has required the "voluntary" or "informed" consent of the subjects. Obtaining consent from the prospective subject serves a variety of purposes, ranging from promoting the individual's autonomy to involving the public in the research enterprise (12). As noted above, respect for persons requires that persons be treated as ends in themselves, not simply as means to an end. Requiring "informed consent" is one way of ensuring that the will of another is respected and that the other is treated as an end and not merely as a means (13).

The Nuremberg Code cites four aspects of valid consent. The subject must: (a) have the "legal capacity" to give consent; (b) be "so situated as to be able to exercise free power of choice;" (c) have "sufficient knowledge" upon which to decide; and (d) have "sufficient . . . comprehension" to make an "enlightened" decision. To the extent that research subjects are not legally competent to consent (e.g., children), are situated in positions of diminished freedom (e.g., prisoners), or are incapable of understanding information given (e.g., mentally retarded persons), or to the extent that the research design requires less than full disclosure of information, the conduct of research appears to violate the principle of respect for persons as expressed in the requirement of "informed consent" (11).

In this regard, the use of institutionalized mental patients in neuropsychopharmacologic research is open to multiple jeopardy. The fact of institutionalization may compromise the freedom of prospective subjects. They may have been judged legally incompetent. Some may not be able to understand information conveyed. And, of course, some neuropsychopharmacologic research requires less than full disclosure of information (e.g., where full disclosure would establish a "placebo effect" in suggestible patients). Thus, one or all of the minimal requirements for "informed consent" may be compromised.

"Free Power of Choice"

Institutionalized mental patients may be legally competent; they may be able to understand information given; and full disclosure may be practiced. Nonetheless, they are institutionalized. What bearing does the very fact of institutionalization have on their power to consent to participate in research? Are they "so situated as to be able to exercise free power of choice?"

The Nuremberg Code prohibits "any element of force . . . or other ulterior form of constraint or coercion" in obtaining consent from a prospective subject (11). A "consent" form signed under threat of punishment for not signing would be invalid. The question is whether other, more subtle forms of "constraint" or "coercion" that may exist in an institution also render consent invalid. Institutionalized patients may be afraid not to "cooperate" with institutional authorities; the possibility of better living conditions in a research unit may entice patients living in restricted, boring conditions (14). Do such circumstances constitute forms of "ulterior constraint or coercion" that would invalidate consent? Many argue that they do.

But these circumstances are not unique to institutionalized persons. Many outpatients are also deeply dependent on doctors and institutions; many poor persons would be "enticed" by better living conditions, relief from boredom, or monetary remuneration for participation. If such factors are to keep persons from participating in research, then we will indeed be reduced to Jonas's proposal that only scientists and researchers are truly qualified to give consent (and only those living in good conditions!).

I would argue that such circumstances do not constitute "coercion" in the strict sense of the Nuremberg Code and therefore do not render consent invalid. "Coercion" consists in a threat to render one's circumstances worse if one does not do something (15). Thus, a threat to withdraw basic necessities of existence or in some other way to make an institutionalized patient's situation worse if he or she declines to participate in research would constitute coercion and render consent invalid. But the provision of better living conditions in exchange for participation in research does not constitute a *threat* to make conditions worse, but only an enticement to make them better. Strictly speaking, therefore, it is not a "threat" or "ulterior constraint" and not "coercion." Similarly, the desire of a patient to "get well" or to impress institutional authorities may be a very real psychological constraint, but is not an "ulterior constraint" in the terms of the Nuremberg Code (11).

Nonetheless, while such enticements do not destroy the *voluntariness* of the patient's choice, they may make choices less than ideally rational—that is, they may prevent patients from choosing the best means to an end by making one means seem so much more desirable than any other. For this reason, most commentators agree that inducements to participate in research should not be overbearing and that, to the extent possible, conditions under which patients are invited to participate in research should approximate those of a free-living or noninstitutionalized person. While institutionalized mental patients may thus be "free" (not coerced) to choose to participate in research, safeguards may be needed to ensure that they enter negotiations for research under relatively fair conditions.

Competence and Comprehension

The current tendency to perceive as "coercive" an increasingly wide range of circumstances reflects an attempt to expand the definition of "coercion" to incorporate not only the "ulterior constraints" of which the Nuremberg Code speaks, but also "interior constraints" such as moods and desires. For example, Ashley proposes: "The lack of freedom arises not only from the lack of information, but also from the emotional factors which inhibit the person" (3). Such an expanded definition of coercion would require assessments of the inner states and motives of patients in order to judge their freedom. Problems with such a requirement are amply reflected in current debates about standards for competence and the link between competence and comprehension.

The Nuremberg Code requires both "legal capacity" to consent and "sufficient understanding" to reach an "enlightened decision" (11). By separating these requirements, it suggests that legal competence need not be based on comprehension. Nonetheless, definitions of competence often incorporate elements of comprehension—the ability to evaluate relevant information (16), to understand the consequences of action (17), and to reach a decision for rational reasons (13, 18).

Goldstein (19) charges that defining competence in terms of comprehension and rational decision making is "pernicious" since a patient's refusal to participate in research where participation would seem the "rational thing to do" might be taken as grounds for an assessment of incompetence! The purpose of the "informed consent" requirement, he argues, is to guarantee the exercise of free choice, not to judge the rationality of the choice. He proposes that competence should be presumed and that, normally, only a "showing that the patient is comatose" should be accepted as proof of incompetence.

Most commentators do not accept such a restrictive definition. But most do agree that such judgments should be limited in several important ways: (a) A judgment of "incompetent" applies only to certain areas of decision making; one can be "incompetent" for purposes of business transactions, but quite "competent" to manage one's personal affairs. (b) Confinement to an institution does not necessarily imply incompetence. (c) Patients can be legally competent (i.e., they have never been adjudicated "incompetent" by court hearing), but functionally incompetent (e.g., they may not communicate with anyone—thus it is impossible to know whether they understand information given); conversely, they may be legally "incompetent," but functionally able to comprehend and act rationally on information given (e.g., many children would fall into this category). (d) Those whose incompetence is intermittent (e.g., due to temporary inebriation or insanity) may need to be treated differently from those whose incompetence is permanent (e.g., some mentally retarded persons) since the former could give consent while competent for participation in research when they are incompetent. (e) Finally, with the exception of children, where the *class* by definition is legally incompetent, judgments about incompetence should be made on an individual basis.

Several of these limitations appear to be contravened by the famous *Kaimowitz* psychosurgery case (20). Since psychosurgery, like the administration of psychotropic drugs, involves mind-altering interventions, any long-lasting effects of this decision will have ramifications for neuropsychopharmacologic research. The decision and its continued interpretation thus merit attention.

The *Kaimowitz* court found that the effects of long-term institutionalization were so destructive of a person's ability to make decisions that, by implication, all persons incarcerated for long periods of time would be automatically "incompetent" to make certain choices—especially those related to participation in irreversible, experimental interventions of unknown risk. If this decision is taken at face value, it might preclude the use of institutionalized patients in research involving experimental interventions with psychopharmacologic agents where the risks were unknown, on grounds that such patients would be by definition "incompetent" to give consent to such research. However, the decision has been severely criticized both because it appears to make a class judgment with respect to incompetence and because it links the very determination of incompetence to the very fact of institutionalization (18, 21, 22). I suspect that this decision will be overturned in time and will not present a threat to the future of neuropsychopharmacologic research on grounds of the incompetence of institutionalized mental patients.

Nonetheless, there are some mental patients who are either legally or functionally incompetent or both. The Nuremberg Code makes no provision for their use as subjects of research.[6] Subsequent codes and discussion have tended to allow their use with certain restrictions: (a) that mentally competent adults are not suitable subjects (24), (b) that the veto of a legally incompetent but minimally comprehending subject is binding (18), and (c) that consent of the legal guardian be obtained (25).

Debate has arisen whether a guardian may give consent for the participa-

---

[6] Ramsey (23) notes, however, that the original draft of the Code included such a provision.

tion of an incompetent person in research not involving any therapeutic interventions. Adopting a "battery" approach, Ramsey (23) argues that the use of nonconsenting subjects is wrong even if no risk is involved, because to use someone without their consent constitutes "wrongful touching." Such "wrongful touching" is rectified only when the research includes therapeutic interventions related to the subject's own recovery.

Yet Ramsey acknowledges that the use of *competent* subjects without their will would not be justified simply because they would be benefited by what is done to them. It will still be "wrongful touching." Why, then, does benefit to the person justify such touching for a child or incompetent adult? McCormick (26) proposes that the validity of such interventions rests on the presumption that the child (and, by analogy, the incompetent adult), if capable, *would* consent to therapeutic interventions. This presumption in turn derives from the general human *obligation* to seek therapy. It is because all humans have an obligation to seek therapy that we can rightly presume that children or incompetent persons *would* consent to therapy if they could and hence that it is permissible to give "proxy consent" on their behalf.

But if this is true, suggests McCormick, then we can also give "proxy consent" for involving children or incompetent adults in other activities where we can presume consent based on their moral obligations as members of the human community. One such obligation is to contribute to the general welfare when such contribution requires little or no sacrifice. Thus, non-consenting subjects may be used in research not directly related to their own benefit as long as the research fulfills an important social need and involves no discernible risk.

One might ask, of course, whether incompetent persons really *do* retain all the normal obligations that accrue to competent adults simply as members of the human community. Freedman (27) argues that children (and perhaps incompetent adults) differ from competent adults in terms of their moral stature and thus in terms of the obligations that can be expected of them. Precisely because this is so, he suggests that the principle of "respect for persons" requires first of all that they be protected, not that their will be respected. Thus, he agrees with McCormick that research is permissible provided that it presents minimal risk, and he rejects Ramsey's use of the "battery" argument.

This debate, as well as the debate over the definition of "incompetent," reflects the underlying tension between the duty to respect the self-determination of others and the duty to protect them from harm, both of which are implied in the principle of "respect for persons." The exact boundaries between allowing individuals to exercise freedom of choice and protecting them from possible harms of their choices have never been adequately enumerated in the arena of research. This is an area where additional work is needed—

particularly as courts struggle with whether there is a "right to treatment" or a "right to refuse treatment."

But, in addition, I would argue that this debate points to a fundamental misunderstanding about the nature of research. As indicated above, "research" is a class of activities designed to contribute to generalizable knowledge through the gathering of data and analysis of data in accordance with scientific principles. Even where this "research"is done on therapeutic interventions (e.g., where two accepted treatment modalities are compared), there are likely to be additional interventions necessary for purposes of research (e.g., drawing blood samples or asking the patients to fill out forms). Most of these interventions present mere inconvenience to subjects. But none of them is primarily intended to benefit the subjects; rather, insofar as they are required for research purposes, they are designed to gather data for purposes of generalizing knowledge. Thus, such interventions, even if done in the context of other "therapeutic" interventions, cannot be justified in terms of "benefit" to the subject.[7]

If the additional interventions necessary for research purposes present risk to the subjects, then it is not clear on what grounds proxy consent for participation in such research should be acceptable even when the research is done around therapeutic interventions. And if proxy consent for participation in research is acceptable in a therapeutic setting because the interventions imposed for research purposes present mere inconvenience to the subjects, then proxy consent for participation should be acceptable in any research that presents no more than mere inconvenience. In condoning proxy consent for "therapeutic" research while condemning proxy consent for "nontherapeutic" research, Ramsey and others appear to equate *research* with *experimental intervention.* Accurate analysis of the moral questions involved is better served by distinguishing between these two. Once again, this is an area where much work is needed. For our purposes, we may simply note that use of institutionalized mental patients in research need not be limited to research on therapeutic interventions even in the case of "incompetent" subjects. What is germane is not whether the research is done on therapeutic interventions, but whether it involves risk.

Disclosure of Information

The Nuremberg Code requires that subjects be told "the nature, duration, and the purpose of the experiment; the method and means by which it is to be conducted; all inconveniences and hazards reasonably to be expected; and

---

[7]The unfortunate tendency to bifurcate research into "therapeutic" and "nontherapeutic" research obscures this fundamental fact and obfuscates moral analysis.

the effects upon [their] health or person which may possibly come" (11). Subsequent codes have modified these requirements, and there is no universal agreement on standards for disclosure—on what is necessary to ensure an "informed" consent. Suggestions range from disclosure of the names of members of the Institutional Review Board (IRB) that approved the research to disclosure of reasons why the particular subject was selected (6, 28).

Among those elements generally accepted as necessary to disclose is the requirement that possible risks be disclosed. But even here there is room for interpretation: Must an investigator disclose an infinitesimal chance of substantial harm? A substantial chance of infinitesimal harm? As Annas et al. (18) succinctly note, "neither the courts nor the legislatures have defined with precision either the quality or probability of the risks that must be disclosed . . . ."

Some pharmacologic agents have long-range, potentially permanent side effects. Where such risks are known, prospective subjects must be informed of them. But, in many cases, we simply do not know what the long-range effects may be. Researchers (and review boards) must be wary of assuming that the risks are small simply because the known and immediate effects are not detrimental, and prospective subjects must be informed of the potential for long-term side effects of a deleterious nature.

Disagreements about the exact data required to render consent "informed" arise in part from shifting standards for the grounds of disclosure: Are requirements for disclosure to be determined by (a) general medical practice or opinion, (b) what a "reasonable" person would require, or (c) the idiosyncrasy of the individual subject? The legal trend appears to be shifting from the first to the second (29). To the extent that the requirement of "informed" consent derives from the duty to respect the self-determination of others, the third standard would seem to be the most appropriate (18, 28). Legally, the requirement would be to give whatever information might be "material" to that person's decision, whether or not physicians in general or "reasonable persons" would require disclosure of that element of information.

But what does one do when the subject requires less than full disclosure— when what is "material" for that subject falls below the standards of the medical community or the reasonable person? Freedman (27) argues that patients or prospective subjects should be allowed to request less than full disclosure—that consent can be valid without being fully informed. But Veatch (28) argues that a person who refuses to accept as much information as a "reasonable person" would require should not be accepted as a subject.

I propose another alternative. When a prospective subject requests nondisclosure, the reasons for that request should be scrutinized. A patient requesting nondisclosure or incomplete disclosure might simply be affirming trust in the physician's judgment. Alternatively, that patient might be expressing a feeling of worthlessness—a sense of "my life is meaningless, so it doesn't matter what they do to me." These two patient-centered reasons are different in morally relevant ways. One is an affirmation of covenant: it affirms the link between patient and physician. The other is a denial of covenant: it denies human relationship by denying the worth of one of the relating parties. Where the covenant is not affirmed, the patient should not be used, because the fundamental identity of the patient's will with the purposes of the research is missing. I would also propose that patients who request nondisclosure should not be used as subjects if there is any doubt as to the root of their motivation for the request.[8]

Nonetheless, there does not seem to be any *a priori* reason why institutionalized mental patients could not give consent to participate in neuropsychopharmacologic research. Provided that they are adequately informed and precautions are taken in cases where they request less than full disclosure, provided that the institutional setting approximates the "free-living state" sufficiently so as not to undermine the rationality of their decision, and provided that either they are competent or proxy consent can be obtained and the research imposes no more than mere inconvenience, their consent to participate is valid.

SPECIAL PROBLEMS IN NEUROPSYCHO-PHARMACOLOGIC RESEARCH

Questions of the justification of research in general, of how to select subjects for research, and of whether institutionalized mental patients can give informed consent are not unique to research in psychopharmacology. They apply to much other research as well.

I would like to turn now to some questions that are more unique to neuropsychopharmacologic research, though once again they may be raised in other contexts as well. These questions have been less adequately addressed in the literature to date, and I shall simply try to suggest the principles relevant to each and possible modes of resolution.

---

[8] I recognize the dangers and weaknesses of a proposal that allows "paternalistic" (or parentalistic) judgments about another's motivations. But I also find from my own experience that turning over decision making to another does not necessarily mean that one has lost autonomy. The proposal intends to respect patients' self-determination while yet protecting them from harm.

Incomplete Disclosure

Questions of incomplete disclosure arise most often not because prospective subjects request less than full disclosure, but either because research design appears to require it (e.g., in order to avoid "placebo effects" from suggestion) or because physicians judge it not in the best interests of a patient who may become a subject. These restrictions on disclosure are likely to arise frequently in neuropsychopharmacologic research, since the purpose of the research is often to assess the effects of pharmacologic agents on mood or feeling (and hence, to suggest possible discomforts involved in the research lends the possibility of "suggestion-induced" discomfort). In addition, the subjects are often patients with volatile and vulnerable mental states who might be harmed by disclosure.

Research designs requiring less than full disclosure should be carefully scrutinized to determine that there is no alternative way to test the hypothesis with more adequate disclosure. If there is not, then the requirement of informed consent (and the principle of "respect for persons" on which it rests) must be balanced with the requirements of good research design and possible benefits from the research. Only research judged to have considerable potential benefit should be allowed. Even so, the benefits from research do not always justify withholding information. Minimally, the principle of "respect for persons" would seem to require that prospective subjects or their proxies be informed that disclosure will be incomplete and that full disclosure is available upon completion of the research. Some advocates have suggested additional mechanisms to provide added protection in instances of incomplete disclosure—for example, consultation with a surrogate or "mock" population to whom complete disclosure could be made prior to entering negotiations with prospective subjects (9).

Professional codes have generally allowed physician-investigators to withhold information that they judged might be harmful to patients—e.g., to withhold from a paranoid patient knowledge that, in addition to the patient's own report of the effects of a drug, his or her every movement will be recorded and analyzed by independent observers. Recent critics charge that invoking the doctrine of "therapeutic privilege" to justify withholding of information from a prospective subject is almost never appropriate since it gives the investigator too much license to serve vested interests by withholding information that might be material to the person's decision (18).

This is another instance where clarifying which interventions are done for *research* purposes and which for *therapeutic* purposes might simplify the matter. Suppose that a study is to be done comparing two drugs used in the treatment of schizophrenia, and that some of the patients to be used as subjects do not know the diagnosis of their condition. Does "informed consent" for participation in research have to include this information, even if the physician judges that it would be harmful to the patient? If that information is not required for "informed consent" to treatment,[9] and if two treatment modalities are to be compared, then "informed consent" for the *research* need deal only with those additional interventions (or changes in treatment) that will be imposed *for research purposes*—e.g., randomization, if necessary, or any changes in diet or activity. In most cases, it will not be necessary to withhold information about the research itself.

But suppose that a new "psychedelic" drug is to be compared to the accepted treatment modality. Here, the fact that a drug is "psychedelic" might be material to the patient's decision about participation, and, if so, that information should not be withheld. If a physician judges it very inadvisable to give such information to a particular patient, that patient should not be invited to participate in the study.

Since incomplete disclosure in such cases is justified on grounds that patients need protection from harm and since patients are deprived of the opportunity to protect themselves by giving or withholding "informed" consent, the research must present no risk to the subjects or there must be special safeguards for their welfare.

The Right to Withdraw

From the Nuremberg Code to the most recent DHEW guidelines, a cardinal tenet of the ethics of research is the requirement that subjects be free to withdraw from the research at any time. This requirement is problematic in neuropsychopharmacologic research for two reasons.

First, subjects are often administered drugs intended to change their mood or mental state. The effect of the drugs may be such as to render them less able to exercise voluntary choice, express their desires, or even display a minimum of self-protective concern. Thus, they may be less able to choose to withdraw (3). Here, it may be possible to negotiate with prospective subjects how they wish their requests and activities while under the influence of drugs to be interpreted and what conditions might constitute grounds for removing them from the study even if they are unable to verbalize such a request. And, of course, when subjects are unable to request withdrawal, the

---

[9] Whether it should be is beyond the scope of this essay. See the essay by Jonsen and Eichelman in this volume.

responsibility of researchers to remove them at signs of danger or harm is greater.

Second, once drugs have been administered, it is not always possible to counteract their effects—one must simply "live through" the experience until the drug has "run its course." Thus, a desire to withdraw simply cannot always be effectuated (31). Prospective subjects must be told of this contingency in the process of negotiating consent. Moreover, prospective subjects should be told what plan of action will be followed should they request withdrawal in such a situation.

The Induction of Psychotomimetic States

Some neuropsychopharmacologic research involves the induction in normal volunteers of psychotomimetic states: "loss of ego boundaries," including distortions of body image and feelings of depersonalization; the impairment of mental function, including incoherence; and the evocation of affectively charged personal experiences (32). Is it ethical to induce such states in normal persons?

Some commentators have argued that it is not unethical to induce such states provided that they are brief: ". . . I would say that it is not an injury to a person to experience *briefly* a condition of derangement or hallucination" (3). The problem here, of course, is that even a brief experience can leave long-lasting emotional effects; thus, the length of the experience itself does not necessarily indicate the harm done to the subject. Moreover, there is always the problem of "flashbacks" occurring in an uncontrolled environment.

Once again, this appears to be a question of balancing the duty to respect the self-determination of others (i.e., the right to consent) against the duty to protect others from harm. The answer to the question depends largely on whether one interprets the principle of "respect for persons" to require primarily respecting the will of another or primarily protecting the other's well-being. I would suggest that it is not antithetical to the meaning of "respect for persons" to offer persons the opportunity to participate in such research, but that this offer should be made only to those persons who are well situated to protect themselves from harm by exercising truly voluntary informed consent.

Consent to Change the Consenting Organ

Closely related to the above question is the question of whether one can morally give consent to have one's "consenting organ" altered.

Some observers claim that one cannot give truly "informed" consent to participate in research with mind-altering drugs because it is simply impossible to understand the implications of altered psychologic functioning (33, 34). In the absence of such understanding, consent might be judged invalid. However, as we have seen above, consent can be valid without being "fully informed."

Even so, some might not consider it morally permissible to give consent to have one's mood, mental state, or behavior altered. These are expressions of the "self" in some sense. Thus, as Breggin puts it, "tampering in the brain . . . must impair the expression of your spiritual self" (35). Or, as another commentator suggests, experiments involving the psyche, of necessity, involve a reduction of free will in that the *person*, rather than simply the use of the person's body, is in some sense placed under the control of the investigator (30). Since people are not allowed to sell themselves into slavery, one could also argue that they have no right to sell their "self" to neuropsychopharmacologic research.

However, this argument appears to make too much of the difference between drugs and other forms of interventions that change the "self"—psychotherapy, psychoanalysis, sex-change operations, and the like. Indeed, enrolling in an educational program may be a way of changing one's self! The limits, if any, on one's freedom to change one's self need further exploration. For the moment, we can say that if participation in research involving psychotherapy or psychoanalysis is not morally forbidden, there appears to be no reason to forbid participation in neuropsychopharmacologic research.

Inducing Addiction

One of the most important but controversial aspects of neuropsychopharmacologic research is testing for the addictive properties of new analgesics. Is it ethical to do such research and, if so, how should it be done?

The answer to the first question is easy: Yes, it is ethical to do such research. Indeed, it would be unethical not to do it since patients might be harmed by the use of nonvalidated drugs.

But there is considerable controversy over who should be the subjects of such research. Until recently, inmate volunteers who were former addicts were used. Their use was justified on grounds that they were best able to comprehend the risks of addiction and thus best able to give "informed" consent.

While it is true that an ability to comprehend the risks of addictions renders former addicts better able to give "informed" consent than most other persons, nonetheless their use as subjects in such research is highly problematic. To begin with, they are prisoners. The voluntariness and rationality of their consent is always suspect because they live in conditions of deprivation and because they are anxious to earn release. But perhaps more important, while they can understand the risks of the research, they cannot identify with its *purposes* (in Jonas's terms). Indeed, the purposes of research appear antithetical to the needs of former addicts whose primary need is to avoid addiction, not to risk it. Thus, I would propose that, in view of the known and serious risks of addiction research, the ideal subjects are those whose needs are consonant with the purposes of the research—namely, patients for whom analgesics are indicated and for whom available analgesics are contraindicated. Harm is minimized by choosing these patients as subjects for addiction research.

Criteria for Assessment

Choosing criteria to measure the success of research presents fundamental ethical dilemmas. As the Group for the Advancement of Psychiatry noted some years ago, value presuppositions affect the choice of a focus for research, the research design, choice of behavior to be observed, and measurements for "improvement" in a patient's condition (36).

The first problem here, as discussed above, is that what is considered a "benefit" by one observer may not be a benefit to another or to the patient-subject. Returning a patient to "normal" functioning may not be a benefit if the "norms" are established by a society whose basic values are not those of the patient.[10]

Another problem is the time frame in which "success" is measured. Administration of a drug may have beneficial effects in the short run, but harmful effects (or no effect) in the long run. More long-range research is needed.

A related question is how "success" is to be measured for interventions intended to *enhance* functioning above the normal state. Research intended to produce "peak experiences," for example, raises difficult questions about what is to be counted as a "peak experience." And, of course, there will be questions about how to set priorities between function-maintaining research and interventions and function-enhancing research and interventions.

In view of the very important value questions involved in the assessment of "success" in neuropsychopharmacologic research, this seems a particularly fruitful area for continued dialogue between the disciplines of ethics and psychopharmacology.

---

[10] Recent feminist critiques of psychiatry have noted the discrepancies between community expectations of women, for example, and true mental health for women.

CONCLUSIONS

This cursory review of some major ethical questions confronting researchers in neuropsychopharmacologic research serves only to demonstrate the need for more probing analysis of fundamental principles and modes of reasoning and of particular dilemmas in neuropsychopharmacologic research. Perhaps most important is the continued interpretation and analysis of the basic principles of respect for persons and distributive justice. I hope the next ten years will see significant work in these areas.

COMMENTARIES

DR. GALLANT: As Dr. Lebacqz has so ably demonstrated, research can be ethically justified on the basis of promoting human creativity and expressing freedom as well as by preventing harm and producing benefits. I agree with Dr. Lebacqz that a system of selection of research subjects which ultimately works to the benefit of the "least advantaged" is a just system (10). However, it is difficult to apply the classical definitions of justice to research. The Marxist philosophy, "From each according to his or her ability, to each according to his or her need," does attempt to protect the weak, but a "straw man" is proposed with the interpretation that the weak, or infirm should participate only in research that provides benefits and no risks. As Dr. Lebacqz infers, such a possibility does not exist. Another extrapolation of the Marxist doctrine to research may be that the seriously ill patient, although not necessarily the "weak" or indigent patient, should be the subject for research associated with his or her specific illness, and not merely utilized for research that has no therapeutic intent; and the benefits of the research should be readily available to him or her. Thus, the two classical formulations cited by Dr. Lebacqz and Rawls's concept of justice (10) can be used as rationalizations for selecting state mental hospital patients as well as other appropriate patient groups for research.

The selection of research subjects is not a difficult ethical problem in those studies with patients in which the potential benefits outweigh the anticipated risks and the scientific methodology is competent. Unfortunately, there are many studies in humans that lack adequate scientific methodology and at times expose the patients to more risks than necessary. At present, the lower economic classes are more frequently chosen to be subjects in research. Moreover, these ward and clinic patients are often the subjects in unfavorable studies where risks exceed benefits to the subject (37). In both the prison populations and lower socioeconomic groups, patient surrogates may be necessary additions to the Human Protection Committees since these two groups are more vulnerable to exploitation than other mentally competent adult populations.

The ethical problem of "Who should be the subject?" may never be satisfactorily answered. For nontherapeutic metabolic research studies, the "semiprofessional" volunteer may be one alternative, according to Earley (38). Earley describes a group of volunteers, housed at no cost in dormitories, paid minimal wages, who apparently select this style of living because they have no desire to work a forty-hour week. This hostelry for live-in subjects is expensive since the subjects can enter and depart the project as they wish. Screening is performed to rule out severe psychiatric disorders and other serious types of medical problems. This is a relatively recent project, and I am quite concerned that this approach might lead to the development of a new type of "skid-row" establishment.

Fried (39) has suggested that new institutions be developed for the conduct of research where a special medical plan might be offered to a certain number of families. A high level of care would be provided in return, with the understanding that these families would be asked to participate in clinical trials. However, I have very strong doubts about the ethics of this type of proposal since it may tend to seduce the poor who cannot afford adequate private medical care. If everyone were guaranteed the right to competent medical treatment, very few individuals would be likely to volunteer for these research institutions since they could obtain competent care elsewhere.

No valid system for equitable distribution of research risks can be devised within our present system. Who among us would be willing to join a lottery which would put us at risk to be selected to participate as research subjects, even if the potential benefits might outweigh the unknown risks? Why not just wait for the potential benefits to develop from the research endeavor while other individuals expose themselves to the risks? Our current society would have to undergo a radical transformation of present values regarding individual rights and obligations to society before an equitable distribution of exposure to research risks would be possible.

Dr. Lebacqz's third major heading was "Informed Consent." There is no doubt that tremendous progress has been made during the past fifteen years in protecting the research subject's right to receive the appropriate information before he agrees to enter a research trial. As recently as 1962, an article in one of the clinical pharmacology journals by a respected investigator revealed his own "personal code" for experimentation performed with certain drugs approved by the FDA (40). This code was a modification of valid consent, and he stated, "I do not always tell patients that they are participating in an experiment." As one of the justifications for this personal code, he cited the possibility that the principal results could be badly distorted if the subject knew an experiment was underway. Interestingly enough, he had preceded this section with a quotation from Kant concerning the unconditional demands of conscience: " 'Every man is to be respected as an absolute man in himself and it is a crime against the dignity that belongs to him as a human being, to use him as a mere means for some external purpose.' " The article was well received, and the "personal code" did not draw any rebuttal or letters to the editor. At that time, the assumed prerogative of the scientist was still unchallenged within the profession and indicated the need for review by outside bodies. Recently, two of the outstanding clinical psychopharmacologists in the world stated: ". . . with many psychiatric patients we feel it both unethical and inhuman to try to obtain informed consent, and we feel that no ethical committees are morally superior to the judgment of the individual researcher" (41). It should be quite obvious to everyone that some type of review of every research protocol for human subjects, particularly in regard to informed consent, has to be performed in a competent manner prior to the initiation of research. All ethical scientists as well as lawyers and laymen would agree that no scientist should do research in a moral vacuum.

Dr. Lebacqz has referred to the problem of incomplete disclosure. In those cases where physicians judge it not in the patient's best interest to give him full information about the study, there is an ethical question of whether or not that person should become a subject in the research project. If that individual is so fragile that full disclosure about his condition would present additional risks to him, then his participation as a research subject is questionable. In those cases of incomplete disclosure that require concealment of the research design to preserve the methodologic requirements of the study, I agree with Dr. Lebacqz that the best approach would require that the subject be informed prior to the initiation of the study that disclosure will be incomplete, but that full information about the methodology will be available upon completion of the project.

The question of how informed any consent truly is may be used by researchers to excuse the deficiencies of their consent forms used in some of their experiments (42). In a series of approximately 1,000 studies reported in American Psychological Association journals, approximately half of the studies were conducted primarily under course requirements, inaccurate information was given in 17 percent of the studies, and only incomplete information was available in 80 percent of the studies. Only half of these studies reported subject debriefing, and considerably fewer reported experiments that did not involve subject deception. If honesty is to exist between the investigator and the subject, then it is imperative to give full information in lay terms to the subject in those studies where foreknowledge of the methodology would not destroy the intent of the study. In those studies where concealment of the methodology is necessary to accomplish the goal of the experiment and where the concealment would be no detriment to the patient during the experiment and/or would not affect his decision to enter the study, written guarantees of full debriefing upon completion of the project should be available on request of the subject.

Loopholes in guidelines and regulations do exist (43, 44). Such statements as "because of inability to communicate" may allow experimentation on seriously ill and even on unconscious people, or "contrary to the best interest" may allow some experimentation on patients unaware of the seriousness of their illness or that is misleading as to the nature of their disease. The question arises whether or not a patient who is too fragile to be exposed to the truth about his illness should ever be used in an experiment. Given these types of loopholes, misinformation about the procedure may occur with approximately 60 percent of those who sign consent (45). A typical misunderstanding found in the survey by Barber (45) was the confusion of the word "new" with "experiment." When told that they were receiving "new" drugs, many of the subjects thought that the investigator meant "better."

Concerning proxy consent for people of limited capacity, I definitely agree with Dr. Lebacqz that the primary question is whether or not the research involves realistic risks and not whether the research is therapeutic or nontherapeutic. McCormick's concept of "reasonableness" contributes to the solution of the ethical problem of proxy consent (46). He has stated, "In other words, proxy consent is morally valid precisely insofar as it is a reasonable presumption of the child's wishes, a construction of what the child would wish, if he could do so." Another guideline for proxy consent is that if the proposed procedure would be objectionable to the mentally competent individual, then it should not be utilized with the person of limited mental capacity.

With these guidelines, it would then follow that subjects with limited capacity to give informed consent could be subjects of research investigations (specifically, neuropsychopharmacologic research in such illnesses as childhood autism, mental retardation, and lipid-storage disease) in which there are no "realistic risks." An additional guideline for proxy consent in research with children is stated in the American Medical Association's Principle of Medical Ethics (24): "Consent, in writing, is given by the legally authorized representative of the subject under circumstances in which an informed and prudent adult would reasonably be expected to volunteer himself or his child as a subject." The Statement of Principles of Ethical Conduct for Neuropsychopharmacologic Research in Human Subjects of the American College of Neuropsychopharmacology (see (Chapter I) offers additional guidelines concerning this very important area of human research.

In the area of neuropsychopharmacologic research, the most common and serious ethical problem that arises in proxy consent relates to research with schizophrenic patients and/or children. Curran has reviewed issues involved in long-term research with particular attention to intervention with children possessing high genetic risk for schizophrenia (47). Since schizophrenia is a serious as well as frequently recurring mental illness, potential benefits from research in this population would be expected to be much greater than from those studies conducted in neurotic populations. It would then follow that the "potential benefits of research for the former population might justify the potentially greater risk of the treatment method and investigation" (47). However, in family and genetic studies of childhood schizophrenia, the actual conduct of the study raises additional ethical questions. Attempts have been made to solve this problem by obtaining clinical assessments of the mental states of both parents to evaluate their capacity to understand informed consent. No family would then be accepted for the study unless at least one parent is capable of giving informed consent. Since research data in these studies might result in the development of prophylactic methods for decreasing the incidence of schizophrenia and possibly preventative treatment for the individual patient, the potential benefits should far outweigh the risks in these studies where the risks may be more than minimal. It has been shown that biologic children of schizophrenics are significantly more likely to acquire the illness than those of nonschizophrenics. Any doubt as to the previous statement has been erased by the adoption studies, adequately reviewed by Crowe (48).

Other vulnerable groups which may require proxy consent in addition to subject consent are the prison populations and lower socioeconomic classes. With prisoners, lack of unimpeded access to information, lack of legal counsel, difficulty in securing objective professional advice, the incentive of the comparatively luxurious research ward, and small financial bonuses help to seduce the prisoner and could exploit him within the research environment. Possibly, with proper Prisoner Protection Committees consisting of appropriate personnel, the prisoner may be able to participate in research studies which offer minimal risk and in some cases specific treatment for the problems that were responsible for his imprisonment. I propose the use of a "patient surrogate" and/or proxy consent for the informed-consent procedure if any one of the following three basic requirements for informed consent are not present: (a) legal capacity to give consent; (b) voluntariness and free choice for consent; and (c) sufficient knowledge and comprehension of the research protocol to make an informed decision.

I would like to address the ethical problem of the physician-researcher conducting research with his patient. Is it possible to maintain the personal doctor-patient relationship with individualized care and yet include this patient in a controlled, randomized study with the physician as principal investigator? In our society, the patient assumes that the doctor will provide the best possible care on an individual basis; therefore, any attempt by the physician to make research participation a prerequisite for treatment is unethical.

In what types of illnesses and with what modes of treatment can research be more easily accomplished in an ethical manner by the physician-researcher? Let me say that those studies that evaluate treatment modalities with the question of efficacy in doubt should be relatively easy to accomplish even after full disclosure about the randomized methodologic procedure has been made. However, in those research projects that evaluate treatment modalities of questionable efficacy but represent great differences in degree of risk, it may be impossible to conduct an ethical study with full information available to the subjects. For example, in the coronary-bypass surgery experiments, if the patients had been allowed a choice between medical and surgical intervention with the full knowledge that superiority of one approach over the other treatment modality was questionable, surely most of the patients would have chosen the medical treatment rather than surgical intervention. This study could never have been accomplished with valid informed consent.

In the clinical trial in which the patient is randomly assigned to one of two or more treatment groups, the inherent features of the doctor-patient relationship are no longer present; this procedure should be adequately explained to the patient prior to obtaining informed consent. Assignment to such a trial removes the personal bond between the patient and the doctor, thus reinforcing the need for an explanation of the experimental methodology. Only in this manner can the physician-researcher be considered to be performing his duties in an ethical manner. If the explanation about the change in the personal relationship of the physician-researcher and the patient is not part of informed consent, then the physician has failed in his obligations to the patient.

In addition to the proper use of local, regional, and national Human Research Committees for review of protocols, specific and immediate steps can be made to improve the ethical conduct of research studies. Specialized training of patient surrogates in combined medical-legal programs is an immediate necessity and should be initiated now. Until a large number of people are trained in this specialized field, either patients' rights will not be fully respected or else research will come to a halt. Other means for improving the ethical conduct of research studies may be taken by editors of scientific journals. Editorial responsibility in these journals has not been fulfilled in regard to the problem of informed consent. There should be a requirement by every medical journal that the article should detail the manner in which informed consent was obtained. I have to disagree with Beecher's recommendation that valuable data improperly obtained should not be published (49). I believe that this procedure in itself might be of questionable ethical value. If we followed Beecher's advice, the patient would have been exposed to experimentation for no purpose at all. It is bad enough to be exposed to research for insufficient reasons, but failure to publish the results would merely compound the error. This procedure would succeed only in masking unethical behavior. Instead, the article should be published and an editorial criticism of the improprieties should accompany the article to expose the author and give some value to the patient's participation by publishing data that may be of help to others.

In regard to improving the ethical conduct of physician-researchers, training in ethics is sadly lacking in medical schools at the present time. Of 350 medical researchers interviewed, only one researcher had had a complete course in medical ethics as a student and 57 percent had never had even one learning experience in research ethics (37). When the 350 researchers were asked, "What three characteristics do you want to know about another researcher before entering into a collaborative relationship with him?" only 6 percent of the replies referred to "ethical concern for research subjects." Of the IRBs surveyed, 34 percent of 293 teaching and nonteaching hospitals had never required any reviews and only 22 percent had members from outside the institution. Continuous monitoring of the projects was almost absent, and, of course, ward and clinic patients from the lower socioeconomic classes were likely to be the research subjects. It is apparent that there are marked defects in the training of physicians in regard to ethical concepts about research and treatment, inadequate screening of review committees, and a fundamental conflict between competent individualized treatment and competent controlled research.

In conclusion, an equitable system for selection of research patients in the future could be developed only if the health care system were reorganized with all citizens participating in the same system. A more realistic possibility at present is the reorganization of the medical school curricula to include the thoughtful teaching of ethical concepts and moral responsibilities in research.

DR. RAFAELSEN: It might interest you to know how it looks from the Scandinavian scene. I will concentrate on informed consent.

Psychiatrists and psychologists have special problems with informed consent for four reasons: (a) They see more clearly the complex aspects of communication between people. They cannot always accept that everything is in good order if only the patient has received, understood, and accepted the information given. In short, it is the problem of rational versus emotional information, and it should not be dealt with as naively and legalistically as is often done these days. (b) They know from experience how stressful it is for some psychiatric patients and their relatives to cope with such decisions. (c) The psychiatric patient is often partially or totally incapable of deciding for himself. (d) At the same time, the relatives too often feel that they are knowledgeable concerning psychiatry in a way that they would never feel about somatic disorders.

I may be able to obtain written informed consent from 95 percent of depressed patients and their relatives to any research plan whatsoever, but even if I could have every member of the legal profession in all countries stand up and applaud, this would in no way solve my own ethical problem: "Do I consider this research plan so safe that I would have my most beloved relatives or myself included in the study?"

I want to call to your attention the 1975 revision of the Declaration of Helsinki (25), which states that certain studies may omit informed consent. Part II, Paragraph 5 states that "the specific reasons for this proposal should be stated in the experimental protocol for transmission to the independent committee." It is my firm opinion that psychiatrists and psychologists should be allowed to utilize this paragraph when it is appropriate and relevant to the research proposal. If they happen to live in countries where this procedure is not permitted, they may use the 1975 Declaration of Helsinki to inform the government and the public that views on this ethical problem vary in different countries. The omission of obtaining informed consent in selective studies has to be ethically justified to the Human Research Committee.

Society wants to stop the evil that may come out of research, but the measures may very well stop the benefits. We will have to go out and tell people what the stakes are. There is still hope that they will realize that it is in their best interests to continue research, not to help us, but to help themselves.

DR. LEVINE: I have already mentioned that the 1975 revision of the Declaration of Helsinki presents us with some very serious problems. Dr. Rafaelsen has quoted one of the Principles contained in Part II, the section having to do with Clinical Research. As I explained before, this is a classification of research that cannot be defined in any meaningful way. Dr. Rafaelsen's comment now draws our attention to another problem with the Declaration. The fact that the reasons for omitting informed consent "should be stated in the experimental protocol for transmission to the independent committee" provides very little reassurance when viewed in relation to Principle I, 2: "The design and performance of each experimental procedure involving human subjects should be clearly formulated in an experimental protocol which should be transmitted to a specially appointed independent committee for *consideration, comment* and *guidance"* (25) (emphasis added). There is no need for committee *approval* called for in the Declaration. You not only don't have to convince the committee of anything, you don't even have to listen to them.

DR. LASAGNA: I would like to express my distaste for the advice given by Dr. Lebacqz. Researchers don't do research primarily for the sake of preventing harm. The traditions of science don't need any apologies for what research has done. It seems to me that the searching for knowledge and information with the intent of doing good, trying to make some order out of the chaos all around us, is a tradition that researchers should not be ashamed of. To follow the advice given here would be a betrayal of our ethics and traditions.

DR. LEBACQZ: I believe Dr. Lasagna has misunderstood me. Limitations of space have not permitted me to detail all of the arguments presented in my essay as justifications for doing research. I certainly do not wish to argue that research does no good, nor would I argue that the good done should not be cited as a justification for the research enterprise.

I am arguing, however, that to justify research *only* on grounds of the good that it can do is to do yourselves an injustice, since it leaves you open to the charge that the good done by the research enterprise is outweighed by the harm that may be done to research subjects. In our culture, the ethical principle "do no harm" (expressed in the medical maxim *primum non nocere)* is generally considered to be the strongest principle. Good that is done for some at the cost of harm to others is not generally considered justifiable.

I am thus suggesting that the *strongest* justification for the research enterprise lies precisely in the fact that it prevents the harm that can result from nonvalidated practice. *In addition to* justifying research on the basis of the good that it does, you can strengthen your argument by justifying research on grounds that it prevents harm.

REFERENCES

1. Swazey, J.P. Myths, muckraking, and hyperactive children. *Hastings Center Report,* 6:16, April, 1976.
2. National Commission for the Protection of Human Subjects of Biomedical and Behavioral Research (NCPHSBBR). The boundaries between biomedical and behavioral research and accepted and routine practice. Draft, Feb., 1976.
3. Ashley, B.M. Ethics of experimenting with persons. In: *Research and the Psychiatric Patient.* J.C. Schoolar and C.M. Gaitz, eds. New York: Brunner/Mazel, 1975.
4. Evans, W.D., and Kline, N.S., eds. *Psychotropic Drugs in the Year 2000: Use By Normal Humans.* Springfield, Ill.:Charles C. Thomas, 1971.
5. Klerman, G.L. Psychotropic hedonism vs. pharmacologic calvinism. *Hastings Center Report,* 2:1, Sept., 1972.
6. Hollister, L.E. The use of psychiatric patients as experimental subjects. In: *Medical, Moral, and Legal Issues in Mental Health Care.* F.J. Ayd, Jr., ed. Baltimore: Williams and Wilkins, 1974.
7. Freedman, A.M., and Itil, T.M. The struggle against irrationalism. In: *Research*

and the Psychiatric Patient. J.C. Schoolar and C.M. Gaitz, eds. New York: Brunner/ Mazel, 1975.

8. Jonas, H. Philosophical reflections on experimenting with human subjects. In: *Experimentation with Human Subjects.* P.A. Freund, ed. New York: George Braziller, 1970, pp. 1-31.

9. Levine, R.J. Appropriate guidelines for the selection of human subjects for participation in biomedical and behavioral research. Prepared for the NCPHSBBR, 1976.

10. Rawls, J. *A Theory of Justice.* Cambridge, Mass.: Harvard University Press, 1971.

11. Nuremberg Code (Judgement on Experimentation without Restriction). *United States v. Karl Brandt,* 1947. In: Katz, J. *Experimentation with Human Beings.* New York: Russell Sage Foundation, 1972, pp. 305-306.

12. Katz, J., and Capron, A.M. *Catastrophic Diseases: Who Decides What?* New York: Russell Sage Foundation, 1975, pp. 82-90.

13. Macklin, R., and Sherwin, S. Experimenting on human subjects: Philosophical perspectives. *Case Western Law Rev.,* 25(3):434, Spring, 1975.

14. Branson, R. Philosophical perspectives on experimentation with prisoners. Prepared for the NCPHSBBR, Feb., 1976.

15. West, C.R. Philosophical perspective on the participation of prisoners in experimental research. Prepared for the NCPHSBBR, Jan., 1976.

16. Shuman, S.I. Patients, subjects and voluntariness. In: *Research and the Psychiatric Patient.* J.C. Schoolar and C.M. Gaitz, eds. New York: Brunner/Mazel, 1975.

17. Katz, J. Human rights and human experimentation. In: *Protection of Human Rights in the Light of Scientific and Technological Progress in Biology and Medicine.* (Proceedings of the 8th Round Table of the Council for International Organizations of Medical Sciences, 1973.) World Health Organization, 1974.

18. Annas, G.J., Glantz, L.H., and Katz, B.F. The law of informed consent to human experimentation. Prepared for the NCPHSBBR, June 1, 1976.

19. Goldstein, J. On the right of the "institutionalized mentally infirm" to consent to or refuse to participate as subjects in biomedical and behavioral research. Prepared for the NCPHSBBR, 1976.

20. *Kaimowitz v. Department of Mental Health of the State of Michigan,* Civ. Op. No. 73-19434 AW (Cir. Ct., Wayne County, Michigan, 1973). This decision was not published officially but may be found in two casebooks: Miller, W., Dawson, R.O., Dix, G.E., and Parnas, R.I. *The Mental Health Process,* 2nd ed. Mineola, N.Y.: New York Foundation Press, 1976, p. 567. And Brooks, A.D. *Law, Psychiatry and the Mental Health System.* Boston: Little, Brown, 1974, p. 902.

21. Mason, J.R. *Kaimowitz v. Department of Mental Health:* A right to be free from experimental psychosurgery? *Boston U. Law Rev.,* 54:301, March, 1974.

22. Medical treatment and human experimentation: Introducing illegality, fraud, duress and incapacity to the doctrine of informed consent. *Rutgers-Camden Law J.,* 6(3):538, Winter, 1975.

23. Ramsey, P. *The Patient as Person.* New Haven: Yale University Press, 1970.

24. AMA Guidelines, 1969. Quoted in: Katz, J. *Experimentation with Human Beings.* New York: Russell Sage Foundation, 1972, p. 485.

25. Declaration of Helsinki. *World Med. J.,* 11:281, 1964. Revised by the 29th World Medical Assembly, Tokyo, Japan, 1975.

26. McCormick, R.A. Proxy consent in the experimentation situation. *Perspect. Biol. Med.,* 18(1):1, Autumn, 1974.

27. Freedman, B. A moral theory of informed consent. *Hastings Center Report,* 5:32, Aug., 1975.

28. Veatch, R.M. Three theories of informed consent: Philosophical foundations and policy implications. Prepared for the NCPHSBBR, Feb., 1976.

29. Curran, W.J. Ethical issues in short term and long term psychiatric research. In: *Medical, Moral, and Legal Issues in Mental Health Care.* F.J. Ayd, Jr., ed. Baltimore: Williams and Wilkins, 1974.

30. Sivadon, P. Experimentation sur l'homme en psychiatrie et en psychologie medicale. In: *Protection of Human Rights in the Light of Scientific and Technological Progress in Biology and Medicine.* (Proceedings of the 8th Round Table of the Council for International Organizations of Medical Sciences, 1973.) World Health Organization, 1974.

31. Inspector General. Use of volunteers in chemical agent research. Department of the Army, March, 1976, pp. 11-17.

32. Cole, J.O., Freedman, A.M., and Friedhoff, A.J. *Psychopathology and Psychopharmacology.* Baltimore: Johns Hopkins University, 1973, pp. 39-40.

33. Dietrich, D.P. Legal implications of psychological research with human subjects. In: *Clinical Investigation in Medicine: Legal, Ethical and Moral Aspects.* Boston: Law-Medicine Institute, Boston University, 1963.

34. Katz, M.M. Ethical issues in the use of human subjects in psychopharmacologic research. *Amer. Psychol.,* 22(5):360, May, 1967.

35. Breggin. Quoted in: Shuman, S.I. The emotional, medical and legal reasons for the special concern about psychosurgery. In: *Medical, Moral, and Legal Issues in Mental Health Care,* F.J. Ayd, Jr., ed. Baltimore: Williams and Wilkins, 1974.

36. Group for the Advancement of Psychiatry. *Psychiatric Research and the Assessment of Change.* Vol. 6 (No. 63), Nov., 1966.

37. Barber, B. Liberalism stops at the laboratory door. Presented at the American Sociologic Association Meeting, San Francisco, Aug., 1975.

38. Earley, K. The subject's freedom: Who is fit for human experimentation? *Sciences,* 19-23, April, 1975.

39. Fried, C. *Medical Experimentation: Personal Integrity and Social Policy.* New York: American Elsevier, 1974.

40. Greiner, T. The ethics of drug research on human subjects. *J. New Drugs,* 2:7-22, 1962.

41. Donald M. Gallant, M.D.: personal communication.

42. Menges, R.S. Openness and honesty v. coercion and deception in psychological research. *Amer. Psychol.,* 1030-1034, 1973.

43. Federal Register-DHEW-PHS. *Protection of Human Subjects: Policies and Procedures.* Vol. 39 (No. 105), May 30, 1974.

44. *The Institutional Guide to DHEW Policy on Protection of Human Subjects.* DHEW Pub. No. 72-102, Dec. 1, 1971.

45. Barber, B. The ethics of experimentation with human subjects. *Scien. Amer.,* 234:35-41, 1976.

46. McCormick, R.A. Experimental Subjects. *JAMA,* 235:2197, 1976.

47. Curran, W.J. Ethical and legal considerations in high risk studies of schizophrenia. *Schizophrenia Bull.,* 10:74-92, 1974.

48. Crowe, R.R. Adoption studies in psychiatry. *Biol. Psychiat.,* 10:353-371, 1975.

49. Beecher, H.K. Ethics in clinical research. *New Eng. J. Med.,* 9:1354-1360, 1966.

CHAPTER V

Ethical Issues in Psychopharmacologic Treatment

ALBERT R. JONSEN AND BURR EICHELMAN

INTRODUCTION

In the earliest days of neuropsychopharmacology, Dr. Fritz Freyhan (1), speaking at the Second International Congress of Psychiatry in 1957, said, "recent years have shown that drugs of quite dissimilar character have been promoted as tranquilizers with the seductive promise of peace of mind for everybody. This has stirred physicians, theologians, and philosophers to make anxious re-examination of therapeutic needs." Twenty years later, physicians, theologians, and philosophers continue their re-examination. Their concerns range widely from the actual and the current, such as the complaint laid before Governor Jerry Brown by former mental patients that the committed are sedated solely for the convenience of their caretakers, to the remote and imaginative, such as Kenneth Clark's suggestion that world leaders be tamed by "antiaggression" drugs. There are concerns that the "tragédie humaine" will be met with chemistry rather than with courage and that children will be shaped not with love and chastisement but with uppers and downers. There are concerns that psychopharmacology will alleviate symptoms and leave untouched the roots of mental disease in personal history and social structures. All these concerns have been entered under the index "ethical issues" of treatment with psychoactive agents.

Concerns over the existence of psychoactive drugs, like those surrounding the existence of nuclear power, seem inevitable, ineradicable, and fundamentally reasonable. Yet, like nuclear power, psychoactive drugs do bring benefits. The therapist sees unreachable patients emerge into human communication. Persons immobilized by depression or broken by anxiety begin to summon their human forces. Distraught patients are eased through crises; distracted children begin to learn. With such manifest benefits and such menacing problems, psychopharmacology is an endeavor permeated with the ethical. As Dr. Laurence Kolb (2) said at the first meeting of this College:

> Your aim is to discover chemical means to modify and control behavior in an attempt to assist the sufferers of mental and emotional disorders to adapt successfully to the social scene. Behavior in this context involves the inherently difficult questions of values . . . values which have determined matters of privacy in regard to many aspects of everyday living.

Of the many ethical issues, we shall attend to certain aspects of the values of privacy to which Dr. Kolb alluded. These aspects center on the difficult problem of informed consent, which we shall examine in light of the ethical principles of respect for persons and justice.

We shall focus on the ethical problems facing those physicians who, after psychiatric training, regularly prescribe and administer antipsychotic, antimanic, and antidepressant drugs in their clinical practice (3). This is a very narrow focus. It excludes the massive problem of prescription of antianxiety drugs by physicians providing primary care (4). It avoids the problems of self-administration of psychotropic agents (5, 6). It only allows a glimpse at the increasing interest in using psychoactive compounds as adjuncts in education (7-11), penology (12-14), geriatrics (15), and espionage (16, 17).

This focus also relegates to the background certain issues which, while undoubtedly important, cannot be explicitly discussed within the scope of this essay. For example, although we are aware that radical critics of psychiatry (18-21) challenge the medical model of mental illness (of which psychopharmacologic treatment is a prime component), we do not discuss their thesis, being satisfied merely to note their warning that, as one commentator states, some "diagnosis and treatment measures in psychiatry are founded on ethical judgments and social demands whose content is sometimes reactionary, often controversial and nearly always left unstated" (18). We recognize that our culture is marked by profound disagreement over the use of mind-altering substances. While clinical application of psychotropic agents might be challenged from that viewpoint (22-28), we refrain from doing so. We are also aware that serious criticisms are aimed at legal, political, and economic institutions that deal with mental illness (29-33). Again, admitting that much of this criticism is just, we only allude briefly to it in our conclusion.

THE ETHICAL ISSUES

Many of the ethical problems in neuropsychopharmacological treatment are the same as those encountered in the practice of medicine generally. Physicians must strive "to do no harm." This implies, in contemporary jargon, a careful assessment of the ratio between benefits and risks. Such an assessment presupposes accurate diagnosis and selection of appropriate therapy. It calls for an estimation of effectiveness and an accounting of the incidence and seriousness of side effects. The literature of neuropsychopharmacology is filled with these admonitions, which are as much ethical imperatives as they are rules of medical practice (34).

It is true that in the early days of psychopharmacology the major ethical problems centered on the evaluation of effectiveness and the assessment of risks and benefits (1, 35, 36). At that time, all therapy was also experimental. Today, to the extent that the search for better drugs and more sophisticated uses continues, the boundaries between research and therapy are blurred (37). The ethical problem of risk-benefit remains a very real one. However, we shall not discuss it for two reasons: first, insofar as it is a problem of research ethics, it is amply discussed in Dr. Lebacqz's paper and others in this volume; second, to the extent that it is a problem of therapeutic ethics, it is not unique to psychopharmacotherapeutics, but is common to all medical practice (38).

Ethical issues more unique to psychopharmacotherapy appear when one turns from the "risk-benefit ratio" to the other constant problem of modern medical ethics—"informed consent." All medical practice has informed consent quandaries: the incompetence of children, the comatose, and the senile; the complexity of scientific information; the anxieties of the patient; and so forth (39, 40). However, in psychiatry, the problem is not acute, but chronic; not sporadic, but endemic. It is the nature of psychiatry to work with patients who suffer from impaired perceptions of themselves and the world. It is an impairment of the "consenting organ" itself which is being treated.

Of course, this has always been the condition of psychiatry: its patients have always been the troubled, the confused, the deranged. However, until the advent of effective psychotropic drugs, treatment was limited to those forms of care that required considerable cooperation, such as psychotherapy, or that were often imposed on the supposedly incompetent, such as commitment, the shock therapies, and psychosurgery. Today, the psychiatrist can draw from the armamentarium of chemical drugs suited for quite particular problems, and varying degrees of mental disorder can be met and managed over varying periods of time. The matter of informed consent appears in a new light.

INFORMED CONSENT

It is axiomatic in modern medical ethics that the actual, implicit, or presumed consent of the patient is the necessary condition for initiating medical treatment. That consent, if actual, should also be informed. This axiom means that patients must assess benefits and risks in light of their own values and that the judgment to which their assessment leads them should be, in the last analysis, the controlling one in initiating, continuing, and terminating treatment (41). How does this axiom apply when patients seem unable to process and organize the information coming to them from the world, including the information offered by the therapist? How does it apply when patients not only seem unable to comprehend, but also adamantly refuse therapy? How can the duty of informing be fulfilled when the information itself may appear to patients as threatening and dangerous? How can consent be free when patients are menaced by their own affectivity, by the threat of confinement, by the pressures of family? It is in this setting of noncomprehension, lack of consent, refusal of consent, and coercion that psychopharmacotherapy is often indicated, as Dr. Stone has discussed in his chapter. Can it be carried out ethically, in accord with the axiom of informed consent? Are there other ethical axioms, such as "to protect and promote the well-being of others besides patients" or "to protect and promote the well-being of the patient," which can be substituted for the axiom of informed consent? These questions, we think, have become major ethical issues in the treatment of patients with antipsychotic, antimanic, and antidepressant drugs.

Unfortunately, the very notion of informed consent distorts the discussion of these problems. Informed consent has become a shibboleth; it is a curt password used by those who would gain entry to ethical territory, but it provides very little ethical information. If "informed consent" is to have any meaning in ethical discourse, it must be interpreted within a more informative and illuminating context of moral values (42, 43). Attempts to use informed consent as a self-sufficient ethical notion are doomed to frustration and circularity; exceptions are sought; fictions, like proxy consent, are created; bureaucratic expedients are devised. Still, the urgent questions remain. While the notion of informed consent now seems firmly planted in the law, we shall attempt in this essay to go beyond it in order to reach more ethically satisfying ground.

Three Therapeutic Situations

1. Frequently patients present themselves to psychiatrists requesting, explicitly or implicitly, to be treated for their mental disorder. An explicit

request is made by overt human communication in word and gesture; an implicit request is manifested by the patient's positing some action, such as arriving at the emergency room, from which it can be readily inferred that help is being sought. Explicit and implicit requests create the happiest ethical situation: the physicians may—some would say ought to—respond, confident that their services are engaged by one in need. On many occasions, physicians can provide extensive information. The patient can comprehend. However, even if it seems that such patients cannot comprehend information about their disorder, its treatments, and their consequences, physicians may proceed in the hope that medication will bring them to a state where such comprehension is possible. It is quite reasonable to consider that the request for help entails consent and that the awareness on the part of the requester that the physician may be able to provide the help is, for the moment, sufficient information.

2. A less happy ethical situation occurs when physicians are faced with patients who neither request nor refuse help (or treatment). Some who seem quite undistressed by their state may be delivered into physicians' hands. Others may be so severely depressed as to be unable to mobilize either consent or refusal. These patients may be mildly interested in the interaction but, at best, passively acquiesce to any manipulation or intervention. Parties other than the patients, such as neighbors, police, and, finally, a psychiatrist, may judge that they need help—a need of which the patients themselves may be unaware. It may be thought that their very need, regardless of the absence of a request, creates a duty to help. On the other hand, it might be suggested that their very helplessness and their defenselessness against others' intrusion into their own satisfactory state imposes an obligation to refrain. At this point, consideration may turn to those others whose concerns have brought the patient to the physician. Do not their concerns deserve a response? Their concerns may range from genuine distress over the retreat of a loved one from human intercourse to bother at the inconvenience of a crazy person in their environment. Still, should these concerns not carry some ethical weight? Should they incline the psychiatrist to treat the nonrefusing, yet unconsenting, patient?

3. The most disturbing ethical situation arises when patients reject treatment. It may be considered that their rejection is but a symptom of their need and that their need gives rise to a duty to treat which overrides their rejection. This was an opinion commonly maintained in the past; today, if still felt by therapists, it is less often voiced. The law has made it quite clear that patients have a legal right to refuse treatment; psychiatrists contradict that right at their own peril. Only the well-founded judgment that patients, as a result of their mental illness, might be dangerous to themselves or to others or that they are gravely disabled justifies overriding patients' refusals. This judgment is often difficult to verify by objective evidence.

This is a distressing situation. In the second case, we may feel justified in overriding lack of consent because of the urgent concerns of others. We are less ready to override refusal. Therapists may have a strong impulse to render aid, which might incline them toward persuasion and, sometimes, even toward deception and coercion "in the best interests of the patient." Use of ethically shady means to this ethically noble end may trouble the conscience of the sensitive therapist. In addition to the impulse to help, the therapist may harbor a suspicion that, should the refusal be honored, the patient would cause harm. Yet, the suspicion may be vague and undemonstrable. In these situations, the inclinations of physicians may be supported not only by the concerns of others, but also by the insistent demands of these others to be protected from or relieved of the patient. Further, some psychiatrists may have a commitment to a private enterprise or to a public agency whose interests they are charged with protecting. The refusing patient may present a threat to those interests. Finally, should the patient be committed, he or she has a legal right to be treated, thus imposing upon the physician a legal duty to treat, as Dr. Stone has discussed in his chapter. Yet, what if the patient continues to resist treatment? Does the physician's legal duty ethically override the patient's refusal? Many currents flow through this situation, rushing strongly to drown out the patient's refusal.

Respect for Persons

How can these ethical situations, particularly the second and the third, be met? In the first, consent, though disguised, is present in the request, but information and its comprehension may be absent. In the second, consent is neither offered nor denied; information and comprehension seem totally lacking. In the third, regardless of information or comprehension, consent is refused. No doctrine of informed consent is strong enough to handle these problems. We must turn, as we said earlier, to an overarching setting of moral values and principles within which the activities of informing, comprehending, and consenting are given some moral meaning. We suggest that the notion of respect for persons serves in large measure for such a setting (44-47).

"This notion of respect," writes philosopher Bernard Williams, "is both complex and unclear" (48). Yet, it is an important, perhaps even a fundamental, ethical notion. In a most general sense, it seems to mean a deliberately adopted attitude whereby we view and treat others as unique selves with their own purposes and plans valuable to them and, at the same time, as self-regulating and responsible beings capable of participating in a community. Put briefly, it means that the physician who adopts this attitude will deal with others as autonomous and responsible. Dealing with them in this way involves a variety of actions: allowing others to do what they will, introducing them by the gentle coercion of education into the community, imposing limits and sanctions, responding to their requests, engaging in debate, cooperating and providing for needs, modifying one's own behavior in view of others' needs and wants, demanding that they contribute to the community, appreciating and rewarding them, and so forth. It should be clear that one can adopt the principle of respect and still be faced with many conflicting courses of action.

One such conflict faces the psychiatrist: If respect for persons implies treating them as autonomous and responsible, how does one respect those who seem incapable of acting autonomously and responsibly? They must be viewed, perhaps, as diminished persons, emerging into, or regressed from, autonomy and responsibility. They may be considered potential persons incapable, in certain respects or at certain times, of acting for themselves and with others (45).

Whatever view one takes, it is essential that the ethics of psychiatry rest upon respect for persons. The natural impulse to flee from irrational persons and the temptation to confine, even destroy, irresponsible persons must be overcome. Pinel overcame it when he struck off the chains at the Bicetre; Freud overcame it when he sought incessantly the familial roots of paralyzing fears and desires. We shall attempt to employ one facet of this ethical notion, so essential to psychiatry, as the key to the puzzle of informed consent. That facet appears when we view the person not only as autonomous and responsible, but also as self-protecting. Persons must be able to devise plans, pursue them, modify them, engage the interest and win the support of others for them—all against the adversity of circumstances, the threats of environment, and the self-interest of others. We call the ability to do this the attribute of self-protection; autonomy and responsibility are contingent upon the ability to mobilize one's inner resources and outer circumstances to attain a goal which others will acknowledge.

Psychotic patients suffer from serious deficits in self-protection: they are prey to bizarre ideation and rampant affectivity; they are oppressed by unrelenting doom. They are incapable of rallying inner strength, and by their strangeness they repel, without wanting to, the proffered support of familiars. They are radically vulnerable. *It is the ultimate act of respect, the principle of psychiatric ethics, to attempt to restore or create self-protection.*

Consent

We shall now look at our three therapeutic situations in the light of respect for persons. In the first situation, respect would suggest that a request deserves a response measured by the request itself, neither falling short of it, nor necessarily going beyond it. The request should be treated as coming from a particular person, neither from someone in general, nor from someone seen only as representative of a type. Responding, then, to the request by undertaking careful diagnosis that should reveal the unique cluster of characteristics that make up this person with this manifestation of disease is the first act of respect. As philosopher Williams says of respect, "each man is owed an effort at identification that he should not be regarded as the surface to which a certain label is applied" (48). In this situation, the request itself is evidence of some ability to protect self: the patient has been able to identify and seek a helper; he or she has been able to articulate, overtly or implicitly, his or her own need. Physicians must verify this knowledge by immediately helpful actions; they are obliged to provide further knowledge only concurrently with the emergence of the patient's ability to add that knowledge to his or her own armamentarium for self-protection. In this situation, the advice of Klein and Davis (49) seems quite appropriate. Discussing how much information about treatment should be given to the patient, they say: "Others . . . feel that it is necessary for the patient to receive all such information. This seems to us to be mechanical. One must minimize the patient's actual risk; causing the patient useless anxiety and increasing the possibility of abandonment of needed treatment seems unjustified."

Lack of Consent

The second situation, in which patients neither consent nor refuse, is not so simple. Such passivity is evidence of a profound deficit in self-protection, which healthy persons manifest either by resistance or cooperation. How does one treat such persons respectfully? Two answers might be given. First, it is respectful to leave them alone and not intrude into their privacy. However, other persons may not allow this course; the state of the patient is for them either a burden, a bother, or a bereavement. They bring the patient to the therapist expecting relief or restoration. A second answer would be that the patient should be treated simply because he or she is human, and to be human means to live in the rational and responsible interaction of a community. Even apart from the request of others or the absence of a request on the part of the prospective patient, treatment is due such persons. Both answers reveal new facets of the problem. The first makes clear the crucial role of others, their wishes and values, in initiating treatment; the second suggests that the retreat of the patient from the human interaction may, in fact, be the only defense he or she can employ against a hostile environment. Should the physician follow the desires of others, the proxies, and risk doing the patient harm by delivering him or her to others who may not take seriously the patient's welfare? Should the physician draw the patient back to interaction, thus thrusting him or her into a world which may objectively be destructive? How does one "do no harm" and "act for the benefit of the patient" in such situations?

Several considerations might be relevant. First, some philosophers suggest that respect may take the form of a "generous love intent on responding to radical deprivation" (44). Such a "love" is not conditioned by consent since it is assumed that consent is impossible. One may assume that severe psychosis is a withdrawal that creates radical deprivation—radical deprivation is defined here to include a loss of awareness of love and caring from others, a sense of isolation and extreme alienation. After observing and diagnosing, the psychiatrist can respond pharmacologically. This will most probably produce results, but only partial ones, from the aspect of "radical deprivation." A complete and sensitive response by the treating physician should be contingent upon an evaluation of the intent of the others who bring the patient and of the circumstances to which the partially healed patient will return. It is conceivable that without additional social intervention the partially healed person will be handed back to those who will not facilitate further healing or that the person will be returned to a world which will undo the healing. These things cannot usually be known with certitude, but often they may be discerned by observation and prudent judgment.

However, is it at any time possible to consider seriously nontreatment of such persons? The drugs are potent and available; the temptation of *furor therapeuticus* is strong. Even more serious, such persons untreated are social problems. Can society tolerate leaving them to themselves, should some therapists judge that their treatment would harm these persons more than help them? We suggest that the answer always turns on the restoration of such persons to a state of self-protection: Can they defend themselves within the community and the environment to which they will be returned? If not, pharmacological treatment may be harmful. Should this be the final ethical judgment, it is incumbent upon society to institute social remedies. There may still be need for sanctuaries.

Refusal

Refusal of therapy creates an even more difficult problem for physicians who are committed to respect for persons. A refusal can be considered an act of self-protection by the patient. He or she repels intrusion into his or her experience. Refusal is the manifestation of one's private being, and it is respectful for others to move away. In recent years, the law has acknowledged that patients have the right to refuse medical treatment, even if this decision will lead to their death or continued disability (50). This right extends to mentally disabled patients. They, too, must accept treatment voluntarily, regardless of others' judgments about their state of mind, as Dr. Stone has discussed in his chapter. Only if they are judged dangerous to themselves or to others or are gravely disabled as a consequence of their mental disorder, as California's pioneer Lanterman-Petrus-Short Act states, can they be committed to an institution against their will.

The current development of the California law seems to conform to the ethical principle of respect: respecting the refusal of the patient who, while disturbed, is not dangerous and overriding the refusal of one who is judged dangerous. This legal interpretation shows respect both for the patient and for others who may be victims of the patient. However, both theoretical and practical problems remain: How is the overriding of refusal for others' safety an act of respect for the patient? How does one judge that another is dangerous? Is it truly respectful to override the refusal of a patient who, though not dangerous, suffers serious illness to the extent of grave disability?

The safety of others may be a compelling motive for restraint; however, its ethical force arises from the awareness that the person restrained is a moral being, that is, a person on whom moral duties are incumbent. First among these duties is the dictum of John Locke (51): "no one ought to harm another in his life, health, liberty or possession." The decision to override refusal is based on a practical judgment that the patient is not, at this time, morally accountable for fulfilling a moral duty. Recognition of the patient as a moral being is an act of respect.

Persons have a duty not to harm others. "Harm" is a broad word, covering a range of behavior from murder and mayhem to the obnoxious and annoying. As one approaches the latter end of the spectrum, it becomes more difficult to affirm a duty not to be obnoxious or not to be bothersome; indeed, one might say that the duty falls upon physicians and caretakers to tolerate the ill. The decision to override refusal of treatment must be justified by strong probability that the patient cannot fulfill the strictest duties "not to do harm." The constant stories of patients unwillingly medicated for the convenience of the staff, other patients, or the family, may represent a desperate response to frustration; they do not display an ethical stance in conformity with respect for persons.

Unquestionably, it is extremely difficult to judge the responsibility of others. It is never a scientific judgment, but always a practical one, requiring information about this person and his or her situation, insight into personality, and the wisdom born of experience. It is, as are all practical judgments, always liable to error. The accuracy of such judgments is a matter for psychiatry; their ethical appropriateness rests on their being made in accord with the principle of respect, that is, by a careful and sympathetic assessment of the state of the person presenting him or herself and by a skeptical evaluation of the claims of others about him or her. It sometimes falls to the least experienced or the least sympathetic to make these judgments. In such cases, both their accuracy and their ethical propriety is questionable. Institutions should be arranged so that such judgments are the responsibility of the most experienced and the most sympathetic.

Further, is it truly respectful to allow a disturbed but nondangerous person to refuse treatment? This is, from the ethical viewpoint, possibly the most difficult to answer. Often, it is apparent that refusal arises from great confusion of mind and emotion. We feel a moral obligation to help such persons toward restoration of their competence. Should an "irrational" refusal be respected in the face of such a moral obligation? Should not all legal means be used to override the refusal?

Klein and Davis, writing of the rebellious adolescent patient, advise that the therapist should become "a reliable individual concerned about the patient's welfare to the degree of overriding the patient's wishes in his best interest" (49). The advice is ethically problematic; indeed, the therapist must be reliable and concerned about patient welfare, but what is the "best interest" of the patient? Certain critics of psychiatry would urge that the best interest of the patient consists in a freedom and autonomy unhindered by others. A refusal represents the most radical act of autonomy and, as such, should be respected. Persons other than the patient, such as therapists, family, or friends, may have no right to subject the patient's refusal to their own tests of rationality (19, 52). However, it can also be argued that the refusing patient, as a moral person, has an obligation to refrain from imposing undue burdens upon others. Persistence in an untreated state may require considerable expenditure of energy, emotion, and money from families or from providers of care. It might be argued that the patient's best interest is, in fact, the observance, under whatever duress is legal, of his or her moral obligation not to impose undue burdens that are avoidable by the acceptance of treatment. This moral argument is plausible, but it is also subject to distortion in which "undue burdens" means "inconvenience" and the "best interest of the patient" becomes a synonym for the interests of others. It is probably this abuse of an otherwise reasonable ethical argument that has led the law to protect the refusing but innocuous patient from therapy. Yet it seems to us that, at least in the abstract, an ethical case can be made in which the overriding refusal may represent an act of respect by viewing the refusing patient as a member, albeit at present irresponsible, of a moral community.

OVERARCHING ETHICAL PROBLEM: RESPONSIBILITY OF THE PSYCHIATRIST

We have attempted to untangle the ethical problems enmeshed in the issue of informed consent. Certain strands were unraveled, but the issue remains a knotty one because it is too closely tied to a larger ethical problem of psychiatry—the responsibility of the psychiatrist. In the medical tradition of Western culture, physicians have been seen as responsible to those who sought their help. Physicians are engaged by patients and are accountable to them. The legal device of malpractice reflects this tradition. Even where physicians were employed by the government or by companies, patients expected doctors to act only in ways that would help them. Physicians have accepted this as integral to their professional ethics (53, 54). The Hippocratic maxim, "I will apply treatment for the benefit of the sick according to my ability and judgment," echoes through the ethics of Western medicine.

Psychiatry is a "medical specialty which," as one textbook author writes, "is a practical way of management, counseling, advice and treatment of troubled, ill, deluded, lost, unhappy people who go to doctors and ask for help. It begins and ends in the patient-physician relationship" (55). To this extent, psychiatry represents the traditions of medicine: the psychiatrist is responsible to the patient. Indeed, during its growth as a medical specialty, it has evolved a most intense form of that relationship and a high sense of that responsibility.

However, psychiatry is unlike medicine in a most significant respect: the decisions of others besides the patient and the well-being of others besides the patient heavily influence the treatment of the patient. The mentally ill person is often incapable of entering and controlling the patient-physician relationship. Others—their families or the authorities—bring them, often resisting, to the physician. The deficits of "informed consent" allow, even require, others to assume prerogatives unusual in the practice of general medicine. Moreover, many mentally ill persons may be considered deviant or dangerous. Communities may find them embarrassing, burdensome, or frightening. Psychiatry, offering to treat the mentally ill, becomes the wished-for social institution which will relieve the community of the presence of the mentally ill, either by curing them or confining them. Psychiatrists, then, are expected by society to act as agents of the community, responsible to it for the management of the mentally ill. All psychiatrists, it may be thought, bear this responsibility; certain psychiatrists who are employed by state hospitals or prisons or are consultants to courts and schools bear it in a particular way. This responsibility to the collective social common good may not always be compatible with responsibility to a particular patient. Thus, a fundamental ethical problem arises: How should psychiatrists fulfill their responsibility to individual patients as well as their responsibility to the community (56)?

Commentators often ask whether the psychiatrist is the agent of society, of certain institutions, or of the patient. In principle, our answer is unequivocal: the psychiatrist is the agent of the patient. The principle underlying this unequivocal answer is precisely respect for persons; it is an act of respect to others to be in fact what one presents oneself to be. In our society, psychiatrists adopt a social role in which they manifest themselves as physicians. That role creates expectations of devotion to the individual patient's well-being. As long as the practice of medicine is understood in that light, it is unethical for physicians, in this case psychiatrists, to perform as double agents. Further, society gives no explicit mandate to physicians to act as agents of society; it does give this mandate to some (e.g., legislators, judges, police) who must manifest themselves as such and who are ethically, if not legally, required to divest themselves of conflicts of interest. Should such a mandate ever be given, it must be circumscribed with the extensive limits imposed presently upon these other officers of society. Finally, psychiatrists may be employed by social institutions that do have the mandate to protect the public interest. Even here, however, the action of the psychiatrists must be unequivocally for the benefit of the patient.

We have earlier emphasized that acting for the benefit of the patient necessarily involves an assessment of the values represented by the concerns of others in the patient's community. *This assessment should be aimed at revealing what is necessary for the patient to return to a state of self-regulation and self-protection. The benefit of the patient is precisely the restoration of these human attributes. Decisions made by psychiatrists which either reduce patients to more abject dependence or take advantage of the present defenselessness of the patient are contrary to the principle of respect.*

However, these questions do bring into view an ethical principle that, while fundamentally complementary to the principle of respect, often seems to contradict it. This is the principle of justice (57-59) of which Dr. Lebacqz has spoken in her chapter on the ethics of experimentation. Respect for persons requires that each person be considered and treated as unique, in terms of his or her own needs and purposes. Justice, at least in one sense of the term, asks about the fair distribution of burdens and benefits within a community of persons with differing needs and accomplishments. Justice is unattainable without respect for persons (60), but the attainment of justice often places limits and even burdens upon some because of the just demands of others. Psychiatrists, presenting themselves in the role of physicians, must adhere closely to the principle of respect for persons and act in ways that are directed to the benefit of patients (rather than proxies) who seek and need their help. However, they are often involved in situations where they must consider the imperatives of justice as well. Acting under the sway of both principles is difficult, for serious practical dilemmas often arise. It is the business of ethics to cast a certain light—namely, ethical principles—and to pose problems within the spectrum of that light; it is not the business of ethics, as such, to resolve the problem, but rather to see whether earnest persons can make practical decisions without moving out of the light of the principles.

Several ethical issues currently agitating psychiatry must be posed in light of the two principles of justice and of respect. The question of absolute confidentiality of psychiatric communication sets the respect due the confiding patient against the interests of other persons and of the society (61-63). The question of cooperation of psychiatrists with institutions of social control—such as courts, police, and prisons—as well as with educational institutions places the need of individuals for personal restorative therapy against the demands of society for order. Both demands, while posed in unique ways for the psychiatric community, contain elements of traditional ethical arguments about the rights of individuals and the interests of society.

It is impossible in the compass of this essay to expound on these difficult problems in the light of justice and respect; we recommend such an exposition to those who will develop a comprehensive ethic of psychiatric care. In conclusion, we wish to highlight one problem confronting those who are engaged in psychopharmacotherapy that evokes questions of respect and justice and that is not often noted in discussions of the ethics of psychiatry. This is the problem of responsibility for the *continuing* care of the mentally ill.

The advent of psychotropic drugs has revised the chronology of psychiatric care. Before the pharmacological era, it was impossible to counter florid psychotic episodes with effective intervention. It was impossible to truncate the course of profound depression except by ECT. It was impossible to respond to debilitating anxiety except by an invitation to enter psychoanalysis. The drugs offer the potential for immediate and effective therapy. Most mental illnesses, however, are not cured by immediate therapy. It is commonly admitted that, at best, symptoms are relieved. Psychoactive drugs, like the antihypertensive drugs, supply an acute intervention for a chronic disease. A chronic disease, however, requires not only medication, but also modification of the environment in which the sufferer must live during and after the exacerbation of his or her illness (64, 65). In the fragmented health care system of the United States, the responsibility of the provider of acute care is not usually linked to that of the provider of long-term care. Psychopharmacologic therapy raises an ethical question about the responsibility the therapist has for the setting of treatment: Does the profession providing acute care bear any responsibility for patients if those patients, once treated, require a particular social setting in which to continue to live in health and comfort?

The drugs may create an illusion that mental illnesses can be treated in a way similar to treatment of infections. Patients treated with antibiotics for upper respiratory infections or dermatitis return to their communities without special problems. Patients treated with phenothiazines or tricyclics must be treated in various settings or returned to a social setting which may be causally related to their disorder. Is it ethical for physicians to deal with symptoms and to ignore the context which may be, in some sense, causative or corroborative of the illness? This problem takes two forms. The first concerns the social setting in which the treatment takes place. It has been noted that the success of drug therapy is closely related to the social environment in which it is administered. Further, the patient's cooperation in therapy must be supported by the treatment setting (66). The second problem concerns the patient released to the community. One of the first benefits ascribed to psychotropic drugs was the return of many committed patients to the community. Subsequent studies have shown both that a high percentage of those released from the hospital are readmitted and that many of those released are lost to needed continuing therapy (67, 68). The existence of drug therapy may have contributed to the disinclination of the government to provide adequate resources for existing institutions for the mentally ill (69).

There are many facets—political, social, and economic—to this problem. Physicians play only a partial role in dealing with mental illness as a social concern. However, their professional judgment on commitment and discharge must be directly related to their professional judgment about the social institutions into and out of which patients issue. This stance should be formulated with consideration of the principles of respect for the person who is a patient and of justice, that is, the fair distribution of the social burdens incurred by mental illness.

CONCLUSION

This essay has focused on current ethical issues in psychopharmacologic treatment. A history of ethical issues would have explored the efforts to determine effectiveness and to deal with adverse effects of medication. A consideration of the future would anticipate, in an imaginative way, the possible applications of psychotropic drugs to a multiplicity of life patterns and problems (70). We found the current issues sufficiently troublesome to feel absolved from the retrospective and prospective tasks. However, we feel that, in one important sense, this essay represents a stage on the journey between the history and the future not so much of the ethical issues as of the ethical methodology. A historical view would reveal that in the early days of psychopharmacotherapy many voiced concerns about the ethical use of psychoactive drugs (71, 72). The questions, while articulately expressed, were not subject to an ethical analysis. This essay attempts to move somewhat further by attempting to analyze the problems in light of the ethical principles of respect and justice. The analysis is, we recognize, rather primitive. We hope that, by putting the ethical concerns into the framework of the ethical principles, future issues will be defined more clearly and debate will center more sharply on the fundamental human values enhanced and endangered by the use of psychoactive drugs in the treatment of mental illness.

COMMENTARIES

REV. McCORMICK: My response to the study of Albert R. Jonsen and Burr Eichelman ought first to state its own limits and lack of pretensions. I comment as a theological ethicist. And by that I mean to highlight my lack of credentials as one with any particular expertise in psychiatry, to say nothing of neuropsychopharmacology. But I mean also, gently, to suggest that theology does have a meaningful word to speak, even if not always a decisive one. Second, as a theologian, I come unabashedly from the Catholic tradition. It is sometimes hard to spell out exactly what that means, even though I am persuaded that how one conceives of and acts upon ethics is profoundly influenced by immersion in that tradition. One of the things I am fairly sure that it means is that I come from a tradition deeply respectful of human insight and reasoning—informed, of course, by faith perspectives, but not replaced by them. I am therefore confident that at least some of my reflections here, if they are properly stated, may be shared.

The Jonsen and Eichelman essay has an importance that goes beyond its individual analyses and conclusions. How we face the very delicate problems raised in their study is paradigmatic. The balance and sensitivity, the discipline and rigor of analysis, the commitment to basic values, yet appropriate tentativeness of formulation, will appear in even more sensitive areas. I believe their essay is rich in these indispensable qualities, and this richness is much more important than any particular suggestions, questions, or quibbling points raised here.

What have Jonsen and Eichelman done? They have taken two[1] of the most difficult consent situations—lack of and refusal of consent—and reapproached them through what they call "the principle of respect." By this, they understand the approach that views and treats others as "autonomous and responsible." They seem to suggest that this is not a fully adequate account of the "principle of respect." *In addition,* they introduce the notion of self-protection—"the ability to mobilize one's inner resources and outer circumstances to attain a goal which others will acknowledge." I say "in addition" because self-protection, if I understand Jonsen and Eichelman correctly, is not an

---

[1] I say two because the first situation that they propose raises fewer problems.

aspect of autonomy and responsibility, but a kind of precondition to their exercise. With the principle of respect so understood—to respect others' autonomy, responsibility, and self-protection—they face the two instances in the following way.

Lack of consent: The patient is presented here by Jonsen and Eichelman as one who is neither dangerous nor imposing undue burdens, but who is a rather helpless, disorganized, and even "crazy" individual. Whether to treat or not to treat is to be solved as follows: "We suggest that the answer always turns on the restoration of such persons to a state of self-protection: Can they defend themselves within the community and the environment to which they will be returned?" The implication here is that if treatment will help the patients more than harm them, and indeed help them in building self-protection, then treatment may or ought to be given. The authors are extremely cautious here, but this is how I understand them.

Here I have some questions for Jonsen and Eichelman. The first concerns the nature of the criterion of "self-protection." To an outsider, this sounds a bit individualistic—as if the community were organized *against* the individual. Why would we not refer to "integration within the community" or "appropriate socialization"? Or again, instead of saying "the ability to mobilize one's inner resources and outer circumstances to attain a goal which others will acknowledge," why would we not say "the ability to devise plans (etc.) in such a way that the goals of others are also acknowledged and respected as one goes about shaping one's own life"? I do not think that this matter is of small significance; for at the heart of the problem we are discussing is the proper balance between autonomy and social responsibility. And if one outlines the problem largely in terms of the value of self-protection, has one perhaps unduly deflated, in advance, social responsibility? In other words, why can we not talk about the *"overall good of the patient"* instead of self-protection?

My second question concerns the description of the "autonomy and responsibility" central to the notion of respect. In describing this, Jonsen and Eichelman refer to treating others "as unique selves . . . and, at the same time, as self-regulating and responsible beings capable of participating in a community." It is the "capable" that could be problematic. What if they are not so capable and will not be after treatment? May we treat them, then, rather "as beings who are part of a community, whether capable of participation or not"? The difference here is potentially enormous. In the first understanding, treatment seems dictated and controlled by its capacity to lead to, bring forth, educe *capability* of participation in community as self-regulating and responsible. The second understanding treats the individual as inserted in a community whether there is any capacity to act in self-regulating fashion or not. If the principle of respect may be reworded in such a way that we ought to treat others for *who they are*—and they *are* social beings, whether accountable or not—then clearly we have a remarkably different criterion, and one that could be the warrant for more psychotropic treatment than the first understanding would allow.

Refusal: Jonsen and Eichelman take two instances of refusal: that of the patient dangerous to self or others and that of the nondangerous patient. As for the first, the authors grant that refusal may be overriden. It is their reason that I find intriguing. They state: "The decision to override refusal is based on a practical judgment that the patient is not, at this time, morally accountable for fulfilling a moral duty." The question that I would like to raise here is with regard to the basis for overriding refusal. There is a long tradition in theological ethics that allows defense of self or others against an *unjust aggressor*—whether that aggressor be personally guilty (accountable) or not. The ethical basis for the permissibility of self-defense is not precisely the innocence or nonaccountability of the aggressor, that is, his lack of responsibility. It is rather the simple fact that his aggression is materially *unjust,* a violation of the rights of others. In this sense, those who are totally incapable of responsible acts (e.g., tiny children) could be materially unjust aggressors and be repelled as such. Or to reword the matter in an opposite direction, even if the person is accountable for what he is doing, we could repel or restrain him. Indeed, the more accountable the person, the more we would *feel* justified in restraining him.

Therefore, if a patient who refuses treatment is going to harm others (in a way that we recognize as a violation of those others' rights) and precisely because the patient was not treated, then it seems to me that this is the radical basis for overriding refusal of treatment. Thus, Jonsen's and Eichelman's discussion of the extreme difficulty of assessing *responsibility* of the patient (who in all likelihood will cause unjust harm to others) strikes me as being beside the point—the point being the root of the moral legitimacy of overriding refusal.

It is here that the principle of respect, as they explain it, seems to get somewhat fuzzy. Why? Jonsen and Eichelman see overriding of refusal as an act of respect for the threatening patient because it contains recognition of the patient as a moral being and "recognition of the patient as a moral being is an act of respect." That is true. But the matter remains ambiguous. Why? Because the term "moral being" can mean at least two things: (a) one who has, as a social being, *objective* duties in justice to others; and (b) one who is capable here and now of fulfilling them, of acting in a morally responsible way. Because they base the overriding of refusal of consent precisely on the fact that the patient *is not acting in an accountable way,* they obscure the sense in which the term "moral being" ought to be understood. They imply that if the patient is accountable—and therefore is one whose unjustly threatening actions stem from ill will—overriding consent would not be morally legitimate, presumably because it would be lacking in respect for the person as a moral being. However, if we take our lead from tradition as it legitimates defense against a personally innocent but objectively unjust aggressor, defense against an accountable but materially unjust aggressor is legitimate. That means that the principle of respect (from the language of Jonsen and Eichelman) is satisfied even when the person is accountable. In other words, it suggests that the satisfaction of the principle of respect in overriding refusal is not tied to accountability primarily, but to the unjust harm to be caused. Or again, it means that the principle of respect relates to "moral beings" understood in the first sense above.

Jonsen and Eichelman conclude this section of their analysis as follows: "their [judgments of responsibility] ethical appropriateness rests on their being made in accord with the principle of respect, that is, by a careful and sympathetic assessment of the state of the person presenting him or herself and by a skeptical evaluation of the claims of others about him or her." That is certainly sound practical advice where the assessment of responsibility is concerned. What I am basically questioning—and that is all—is the ultimate relevance of responsibility to the decision to override refusal.

The point becomes even clearer when Jonsen and Eichelman turn to the refusing patient who is not dangerous. They give two positions, but opt for the second. The first maintains that the refusal of treatment ought to be respected. Others have "no right to subject the patient's refusal to their own tests of rationality." The second position argues that the patient's best interest is actually served by "the observance, under whatever duress is legal, of his or her moral obligation not to impose undue burdens that are avoidable by the acceptance of treatment." Their reason for regarding this as a "reasonable ethical argument" is as follows: "overriding refusal may represent an act of respect by viewing the refusing patient *as a member,* albeit at present irresponsible, *of a moral community"* (emphasis added).

I personally agree with the direction of this second judgment, and I think the Jonsen and Eichelman warning that the judgment is subject to distortion is correct and important. Why? For one reason, it is more difficult to determine what is an *undue burden* than it is to determine what is an *unjust action.* However, it is to be noted that the burden of the analysis falls on objective membership in a community of persons, persons who are mutually interdependent and who have reciprocal obligations in the objective order (e.g., "not to impose undue burdens that are avoidable by the acceptance of treatment"). The weight of the argument is found in the objectivity of the social order, of the social insertion of the patient—whether that person is presently accountable or not or may be made such. This raises the following question: If refusal of consent can be overridden here (where the patient is not dangerous, but if left untreated will impose undue burdens on others) and precisely on the grounds that the patient is a social being with objective obligations, then why is the emphasis on *responsibility* and *accountability* when we are dealing with the dangerous patient, an even clearer case?

I am suggesting, therefore, that since the basis for intervention in the two instances of lack of consent and refusal of consent seems somewhat unresolved and ambiguous, so, too, the principle of respect, which is said to validate intervention, needs clarification. Indeed, one has to wonder whether the principle of respect is a true principle—a source of *derivation*—if its grounds are so remarkably different in the two instances under discussion. Is it, perhaps, adventitious—a way of formulating and summarizing what the authors have actually concluded on other grounds?

There is another aspect of the Jonsen and Eichelman study which I would like to question. After stating the three general case-categories they would like to treat (lack of comprehension, lack of consent, refusal of consent), they state: "No doctrine of informed consent is strong enough to handle these problems." As that phrase "doctrine of informed consent" is ordinarily understood, Jonsen and Eichelman are certainly correct for the simple reason that their solutions at some point dispense with the consent requirement. But their own analysis—even with the ambiguities attended to above— which overrides lack of consent and refusal in certain instances, leads one to believe that the doctrine of informed consent is not adequately understood unless it is carried beyond consent protocols to its deeper analytic rootage.

A brief outline of this analytic rootage may be of help here. The professional requirement of informed consent in medical practice in general is based on (or so I would argue) the *moral* right to privacy or self-determination (I understand the two synonymously). As I understand the moral tradition largely responsible for the elaboration of the consent requirement, the so-called right to privacy or self-determination in health care originates through the following steps (73):

1. Human life, as a gift of God and the condition of all other achievements, is a basic good. Our flourishing both as individuals and as a society depends on the adequacy of our attitudes and actions with regard to this basic good. Any number of more specific modes of obligation spell out the meaning of "adequacy of our attitudes and actions."

2. An individual has the primary obligation to preserve this basic good in him or herself, to preserve his or her own life. The first and most obvious reason for this is that it is his or her life, his or her good at stake. If this obligation did not fall primarily on the individual, how could we ascribe any other obligation to him or her? Furthermore, the individual is the only one who can most of the time take the steps to preserve life and avoid those

things that threaten life. Thus, it is the individual who is primarily charged with feeding him or herself properly, clothing him or herself, avoiding unjustifiable dangers, recognizing threatening disease processes, and seeking remedies. If this duty were not the individual's primarily, who else would do it? (I say "primarily" because it is clear that, as social and dependent beings, we do depend on others in securing our own well-being.)

3. This obligation to preserve one's life and care for one's health is a *limited* one in Christian perspective. For instance, Christian convictions have never allowed one to do something immoral to preserve one's life. There are also limitations where there is no question of immoral conduct. Not all means must be used, otherwise we would convert life from a basic value to an absolute and unconditioned one and, in the process, subvert some profound Christian convictions about the meaning of life.

4. The limits on one's duty to preserve life are very relative to time, locale, personal biography, personal position, personal perspectives, outlooks, achievements, and recovery prospects.

5. The person himself or herself—or in case of incompetence, those closest to him or her—has the best knowledge or understanding of these personal considerations. The individual has the best knowledge of what may be called a "reasonable benefit" to the patient or of what may be too much of a burden to him or her, all things considered.

6. Therefore, one has the *right* to those means that make personal execution of this duty possible and to those means that best provide for the practical admission of limits on this duty.

7. But self-determination with regard to means of preserving life and health is a necessary means.

In summary, as I read the tradition from which I come, there is first a *duty* to preserve one's life and health and, following on that, a *right* not to be interfered with in making moral decisions with regard to this duty. The right of privacy or self-determination is a necessary means because, given the personal character of the situations that activate this duty, and given the personal or individual character of the considerations that limit this duty, it is the person himself or herself who is best situated to implement decisions. This suggests that the underlying supposition for self-determination in the acceptance or refusal of treatment is that the *overall good of the patient will best be served* if treatment is controlled in this way.

Perhaps we could summarize as follows. A moral right is always with regard to a good. The good in question is self-determination in the acceptance or rejection of medical treatment. This self-determination or privacy is a conditional or instrumental good, that is, it is a good precisely insofar as it is the instrument whereby the best interests of the patient are served by it.

If, for example, the best overall good of patients would be better achieved without self-determination, it would be senseless to speak of self-determination as a right.

By putting the matter in this way, namely, by seeing the good underlying the right of privacy as the *overall good of the patient*, we see two immediate limitations on this right. First, when the exercise of this right is *de facto* and in the circumstances no longer to the overall good of the person involved, then the very reason for self-determination or privacy has disappeared. For example, if the person is going to exercise self-determination in a way commonly regarded as destructive to self, then the underlying good which founds the right no longer supports it. The right has met its limits. Or at least at this point self-determination ceases to be an instrumental good. I hasten to add that this is the *moral* tradition. It is probably not altogether identical with the *law* on the matter.

Second, self-determination as a means to the overall good of the person or patient says nothing about the exercise of this right to the detriment of others. That is another judgment altogether—that is, how the overall good of the patient is related to and perhaps limited by the good of other patients is simply not to be derived from the notion of privacy itself. Indeed, the moral tradition would insist that the right in question, like most rights, is not absolute. It is limited by social insertion or membership in a community of persons with their own rights. This may be rendered by saying that the *overall good of the patient* is not to be determined individualistically. Or even more concretely, we may say that if an individual's actions are going to cause *unjust* harm or *undue* burdens to others, they are not to the *overall good of the patient* himself or herself.

That is, I believe, the *moral* tradition on the right to self-determination. It is an instrumental right in service of a subordinate to a good—*the best interests of the person.*

The upshot of these reflections is, I believe, that it is theoretically (at the level of theoretical moral principle) morally justifiable to intervene at times without consent or even against refusal of consent. I have suggested that the basis of this conclusion—a conclusion shared by Jonsen and Eichelman—remains somewhat ambiguous in their presentation. I have further suggested that I believe that the basis is the *overall good of the patient.* This good cannot be delineated in an individualistic way, a point made clear by Jonsen and Eichelman when they speak of persons as "members of a moral community," that is, whose very sociality defines their good and rights, but also limits them. In defining these rights we are, of course, always in danger of tipping the delicate balance between the individual and the community. But such a danger suggests caution, not paralysis.

Above, I used the term "theoretically morally justifiable." That brings me to another observation. The use of such phraseology is designed to underline two things. First, to say that something is *theoretically* justifiable does not preclude the possibility that *practically* it may not be. In other words, there may be reasons of a very practical kind (e.g., danger of abuse) that lead to a prohibitive policy. For instance, one might argue that the cultural pendulum in the United States has swung to an extreme. We are corporately *homo technologicus* and this leads us to an intensely interventionist posture in facing our human problems. Instead of adapting the environment to the needs of underprivileged individuals, we tend to do just the opposite—to bend the individual to the demands of the environment in a way that is uncritical of the cultural environment. Sometimes we do this even to the point of eliminating the individual.

This is all too often clear in our treatment of "defective" persons, especially the retarded, and most especially children. Similarly, we face the aging problem by isolating our elderly citizens in leisure worlds, thinking we have solved a *human* problem by providing certain material benefits. In another area, the solution of the problem of environmental pollution—brought on by technology—is more technology. Further still, in the realm of reproduction, ethicist Joseph Fletcher (74) writes: "Man is a maker and a selector and a designer, and the more rationally contrived and deliberate anything is, the more human it is." Thus he concludes: "Laboratory reproduction is radically human compared to conception by ordinary heterosexual intercourse. It is willed, chosen, purposed and controlled, and surely these are among the traits that distinguish *Homo sapiens* from others in the animal genus . . . coital reproduction is, therefore, less human than laboratory reproduction." And so on.

Now it can be argued that such cultural shadings affect all of us. They constitute the atmosphere in which we think and act. In *such* an atmosphere—which I have called "interventionist"—it could be argued that we must take counterbalancing steps. If the concrete manifestation of this interventionist bias in the field of neuropsychopharmacology is a certain *furor therapeuticus,* then one might conclude that what is theoretically justifiable might not be, all things considered, practically so. I raise this point for your consideration and perhaps enlightened disagreement.

For instance, I am terribly frightened at my own arguments justifying as a *rare* exception the sterilization of a retarded person for that person's own protection and good—frightened where and because I see thousands of poor blacks in the South sterilized, sometimes with appeal to just such arguments. If that is the atmosphere in which a theoretical argument exists, it may never be prudent to reduce it to practice—or eventually even to make the argument.

The second point highlighted by the usage "theoretically justifiable" is the fact that such a statement does not spell out the concrete conditions and circumstances that comprise the overall good of the patient in an individual case. Put differently, such usage does not solve a particular problem; it only prepares for a concrete solution. In others words, it creates the *possibility* of a solution by stating the general perspectives that ought to guide us in the individual circumstances of the particular case. We need more particularized guidelines in the field of neuropsychopharmacology, just as we do in all other areas of human action. But these guidelines are, I believe, your task as specialists. And I believe that Jonsen and Eichelman have provided some excellent considerations and cautions toward completing that task in a human and realistic way.

DR. GALLANT: Rawls has written: "Justice is the first virtue of social situations, as truth is of systems of thought" (58). Social justice should guarantee every citizen the equal right to survive. Competent medical care has to be included as part of this obligation of society to its citizens. In the field of medical care, including psychopharmacologic therapy as well as other psychiatric therapies, the patient's medical rights should include the right to receive honest information, the right of free choice, the right of physician confidence, and the right to be treated with dignity. The right within this context would be defined as the demand that an individual makes on his social system and this demand must be responded to by the system, the physician being the instrument of the social system in this particular case. If one of the ethical values of a just society is to help to preserve life as well as to procreate and preserve the human species, then the right to competent medical care has to be recognized as one of the basic requirements of this society.

The first ethical step toward securing competent medical care requires primary therapeutic intent from the physician. The second step is the patient's evaluation of the benefits and risks of the treatment modality or having the essential information about the available treatment modalities prior to giving consent to treatment. To secure competent medical treatment, informed consent is the basic prerequisite. Without informed consent, no psychopharmacologic interaction can be justified. Informed consent should not be determined by applying the standards of a reasonable medical practitioner in the same locality; rather, it should be determined by applying the standards of a reasonable man and what he would expect to have explained to him. In the field of psychiatry, however, particularly in regard to those patients entering mental hospitals, as emphasized by Jonsen and Eichelman, informed consent becomes a much more difficult and complicated problem. In a study by Olin and Olin (75), only 8 of 100 patients admitted to a mental hospital were considered to have adequate understanding of the terms of the voluntary admission application they signed at the time of entering the hospital. The finding that few voluntary patients are fully informed to give consent to hospitalization poses a problem in view of the trend toward giving personal responsibility to the patient. Schizophrenic patients and patients with an organic mental syndrome, as expected, showed the poorest comprehension.

Another problem arises in association with the above difficulty with informed consent. How can routine medical decisions with mentally incompetent patients be effected without frequent challenges by courts? Is the family or a court-appointed lawyer, possibly inexperienced in treatment modalities, qualified to give informed consent? It should be apparent that professional patient surrogates will have to be trained in medical-legal aspects of informed consent as well as exposed to experiences and scientific knowledge associated with the multiple psychiatric treatment modalities available to patients. In those cases defined as emergency situations, routine medical decisions would be surveyed by the patient surrogate, hopefully utilizing the "notion of respect" as formulated by Jonsen and Eichelman. While the trained patient surrogate could render opinions on unusual treatment problems requiring immediate attention, the decision for maintaining the treatment initiated should be reviewed by a Treatment Review Committee or a Patient Monitoring Committee. Permanent local and regional Treatment Review Committees will have to be established in the future with the patient surrogate as permanent chairman; the ad hoc members would consist of closest family member, family clergyman if appropriate, family physician if available, and a specialist in the field of medicine associated with the patient's illness. The common goal that the patient surrogate and the Committee should seek is that the treatment techniques imposed will produce beneficial changes that the patient might have sought if he were mentally able to give valid informed consent. Although, in fact, this goal is impossible to attain, the attitude stated should be behind every decision made by the patient surrogate and the Committee.

Of course, the citizen-patient has the alternative right not to be treated. If a patient who is not declared legally incompetent does not want to be subjected to any particular therapy, his judgment should be honored. If the patient is dangerous to himself or to others, then it may be legally acceptable to force treatment on this patient with the consent of his legal representative or by a court of law if there is a reasonable probability that the treatment would be beneficial and if the patient is incompetent to comprehend the effects of the therapy (76). Although this concept has been legally accepted by the courts in the *Winters v. Miller* case (76), it is still an important unresolved ethical question at the present time. The "notion of respect" as presented by the authors of this chapter would appear to offer valuable guidelines for such difficult problems.

It has been proposed that any treatment recommendation for nonconsenting patients involving brain surgery, electroconvulsive therapy, prolonged use of tranquilizers, or physically aversive techniques be reviewed and approved by a monitoring agency (77). It must be emphasized, however, that undue delay of treatment may be harmful for the long-term as well as short-term prognosis of the patient. It would be most unfortunate if committees to ensure rights and benefits of patients became impediments to personal care and individualized therapy. Yet accountability is needed and is proper within the context of both research and medical practice by even the more conscientious physician. Although it is recognized that it would be impossible for Treatment Review Committees to review or even be aware of all treatment problems, the very existence of these Committees would serve as a deterrent for the negligent therapist and would foster a more cautious, thoughtful attitude in all who are involved in treating patients. Since prolonged psychopharmacologic therapy can cause long-term side effects such as tardive dyskinesia, and since there are hundreds of thousands of patients receiving these compounds for relatively long periods of time, the existence of these Committees can actually serve as a useful reminder to those physicians involved in treating large numbers of patients.

Another problem, raised by the authors of this chapter, concerns the responsibility of the psychiatrist as an agent of the patient both for his acute treatment and community adjustment. It is sometimes beyond the administrative ability of the treating physician to ascertain whether or not the patient he treated during the acute phase of the illness is receiving satisfactory long-term, follow-up treatment. The structure of society directly affects the type of medical care system within that society, and the physician is only one part of medical care services. In this country we have several different types of medical care delivery systems which may be placed within the two large categories of public and private care. As long as there are two such distinct delivery systems of medical care, it should be apparent that adequate psychiatric treatment of the lower socioeconomic classes will not become a reality in the near future. Ten years ago it was noted that relatively few and inadequate services had been provided for institutionalized patients in state or city mental hospitals to help them maintain their ties to family and community (78). In this country the state and city mental health programs have always been responsible for the treatment of patients from the lower socioeconomic classes. Thus, it is this patient who is more or less neglected by the service agencies of the community. Basic to the neglect is the assumption that the psychiatric patient is the responsibility of the hospital and not of the community from which he came. It has been stated that the community "must join the hospital in sharing responsibility for the care of the patients. A centralized service agency, designated to coordinate all rehabilitative services, should be initiated as a clearing house for referrals and maintain a follow-up on all cases" (78). This advice, made by many different individuals more than a decade ago, has still not been utilized in most communities. Such an arrangement would be an invaluable aid for the psychiatric patient and would help to alleviate many inadequacies in present community services for the lower socioeconomic classes. However, no significant changes have occurred in this area despite all of the monies invested by the federal government. If an equitable distribution of psychiatric services as well as competent medical services to all of the population is an ethical goal of society, thus granting its citizens an equal right to survive, then it may well be that a single system of health care might be more able to accomplish this goal than the two separate and distinct medical care systems that presently exist in the country. If this supposition is valid, then all mental health professionals are obligated to help accomplish the goal of providing an equitable "setting of treatment" for all patients.

Unfortunately, man's ability to identify himself as a separate entity within his species and his ability to initiate an interruption of conditioned responses required for survival of the species to obtain his own selfish ends does raise the question of whether or not the above goal is attainable. His ability to separate himself from the herd and be primarily concerned with his own existence may make it impossible for him to feel consistent allegiance to and to sustain his ethical obligations to society. The pessimist might speculate that this existential dilemma will eventually result in an inhibition of further progress of society. The optimist may predict that man's instincts for individual survival may lead him to the conclusion that equal distribution of justice for the group may offer greater security for the individual.

Ethical issues in treatment should include consideration of the question: "What is the competent practice of treatment?" Thus, I do think it appropriate to define what I consider the competent practice of psychopharmacologic treatment as a starting point for future discussions. The competent practice of psychopharmacologic treatment should utilize treatment approaches that are based on scientifically valid experiments that indicate the efficacy and known risks of the medication administered to the patient. The following information should always be considered before initiating treatment: (a) diagnosis, symptom profile, and possible etiology of the disease; (b) course and history of the disease; (c) treatment of choice; (d) anticipated beneficial effects and side effects of the medication to be used, based on valid scientific research results; (e) alternative treatment techniques available for the disease; (f) concept of duration of required drug therapy; and (g) subsequent treatment approaches if the present medication regimen fails. All of this information should be freely available to the patient or, in the case of mental incompetency, the closest living relative of the patient.

To enhance proper professional conduct in the delivery of competent medical treatment, Jonsen and Hellegers (79) have recommended additional requirements that should be a part of the value system of physicians, such as "a statement about professional character or virtue, right action or duty, and concern for the common good or social justice. . . ." The thrust of these requirements is that no matter how good or pure the social structure or medical care system is, the final and essential basis of competent and personal delivery of medical care to the patient depends on the character of the individual physician who is performing this service. As has been inferred elsewhere in this volume, regulations and law may encourage adherence to professional ethics, but the attainment of ethical goals depends more on the personal character of the treating physician than on legal sanctions. There is no doubt that the teaching of ethics and ethical conduct in medical schools is grossly lacking (80). Neither the federal nor the state governments should provide any financial support to those medical schools that do not offer well-organized courses in ethical problems and conduct of medical research and treatment. Although it is quite likely that most medical students have formulated their value systems before entering medical school, it is still the duty of the medical schools to expose the students to the concepts of right action, duty, and concern for their fellow humans.

MR. FORCE: Consent of the patient or research subject has figured prominently in many of the papers and commentaries. The last paper and commentaries are no exception. All of the papers and comments, however, reveal the limitations in placing too much emphasis on "consent" as the sole legal or ethical guideline in psychopharmacologic treatment or research.

Historically, as an evolution from the "battery" notion, and more recently under the aegis of "privacy" and the First Amendment, the requirement for consent has proved a useful factor in evaluating permissible medical and scientific practices. However, in discussions of psychopharmacologic treatment, the focus on the consent factor alone is clearly a mistake. The simple proposition that medical treatment without consent, real or implied, is unlawful or unethical is only of limited utility in dealing with patients suffering from various mental diseases or defects.

In patients suffering from nonmental physical conditions, the capacity of the individual to understand his condition and proposed treatment is ordinarily assumed, and his consent to treatment is a paramount factor in establishing the legality of the treatment process. Consent in the legal and ethical sense presupposes understanding and rationality. In law, we have qualified the expression so that it is referred to as "informed consent," which means that the patient has sufficient information and capacity for understanding to make an informed decision. The legal requirement is premised on the notion that the information is necessary to an intelligent and rational decision.

Psychopharmacologic treatment may involve situations in which we cannot be certain whether consent is being given or withheld. The patient may be saying "yes" or "no" or nothing, but there may be a realistic doubt as to whether he understands his condition and proffered treatment so as to be able to make an intelligent and rational decision. This is not to suggest that everyone pharmacologically treated for mental and emotional conditions is incapable of making intelligent and rational decisions about proffered treatment modalities. Yet it is undoubtedly true that there exist sufficient cases in which this is true.

The authors of and commentators on this final paper have discussed, among other things, when lack of consent may *not* be the controlling factor in evaluating the ethics of treatment. Presumably, there are also situations in which the existence of "consent" would not, under the circumstances, be the controlling factor in evaluating the ethics of treatment. In this regard, law should follow ethics, i.e., in certain situations, factors other than consent of the patient should control the legality of the treatment. By introducing the "proxy-consent" device whether from a member of the family, legal guardian, judge, or patient surrogate, we have shifted the emphasis away from those considerations that underlie the consent factor—for example, what does the patient want, what treatment will he accept? Where the patient truly lacks the capacity to consent, the "proxy-consent" device or any other legal requirement must not only serve as a barrier to prevent taking advantage of any person unable to make judgments affecting his or her own welfare, but also focus on considerations such as the "overall good of the patient." In fact, it probably would be a good idea to abandon the term "proxy consent" altogether.

The discussion of ethics reveals that in some cases factors other than consent should control the decision to treat or not. The law should embrace those factors in properly formulated legal standards.

DR. EICHELMAN: I would like to make a few brief comments. Dr. Jonsen and I appreciate Father McCormick's comments on our paper; I think that he does hone in on areas of fuzziness. I do want to underscore the term "self-protection" and, in fact, emphasize that we *are* talking about the individual's dialogue and integration with society, as well as his autonomy. I don't think we are really at issue with the comments made by Father McCormick.

Concerning the overriding of consent and psychiatry's intervention in the process of an individual's dialogue and integration with society, we focused particularly on the person who is not perceived as morally responsible. Many persons who are acting irresponsibly, but are adjudged capable of moral responsibility (whose consenting and effecting organs are not diseased), should fall within the jurisdiction of social agencies other than psychiatry.

I do not believe that psychiatry is really prepared to take on the latter group of persons.

I would like to add one more brief reflection. As Dr. Lebacqz has pointed out in her paper, the dialogue on ethics has increased during the past ten years. It has now grown to become the substance of panel discussions and programs such as the symposium documented in this volume. I think we are now beginning to articulate what are the principles by which we should govern and steer, where we should affix our sights and begin to engage in the dialogue of how those different issues of justice and respect for a person should be balanced, and how those issues should be reflected in the law and the legal system. I think that these advances warrant some optimism concerning the progress of ethical research and treatment during the next ten years.

REFERENCES

1. Freyhan, F. In: *Psychopharmacological Frontiers*. N. Kline, ed. (Proceedings of the 2nd International Congress of Psychiatry.) Boston: Little, Brown, 1959, p. 7.
2. Kolb, L. The current problems of research involving human beings: The curse of the Holy Grail. In: *Psychopharmacology: A Review of Progress 1957-1967*. Daniel H. Efron, ed. Washington, D.C.: Public Health Service Publication, 1968, p. 326.
3. Hollister, L. *Clinical Use of Psychotherapeutic Drugs*. Springfield, Ill.: Charles C. Thomas, 1973.
4. Ruth Cooperstock, Ed., *Social Aspects of the Medical Use of Psychotropic Drugs*. Toronto: Alcoholism and Drug Addiction Research Foundation, 1973.
5. Chambers, C., et al. *Chemical Coping: A Report on Legal Drug Use in the United States*. New York: Spectrum Books, 1975.
6. J.R. Russo, ed. *Amphetamine Abuse*, Springfield, Ill.: Charles C. Thomas, 1968.
7. Eisenberg, L. Principles of drug therapy in child psychiatry with special reference to stimulant drugs. *Amer. J. Orthopsychiat.*, 41 (3):371-379, 1971.
8. Fish, B. Drugs in hyperkinesis. *Arch. Gen. Psychiat.*, 25:192-203, 1971.
9. Sroufe, L.A., and Stewart, M. Treating problem children with stimulant drugs. *New Eng. J. Med.*, 289:407-413, 1973.
10. Wender, P.H. The case of MBD. *Hastings Center Report*, 2(1):94-102, 1974.
11. Wender, P.H. *Minimal Brain Dysfunction in Children*. New York: Wiley Interscience, 1971.
12. Resnick, O. Use of psychotropic drugs with criminals. In: *Psychotropic Drugs in the Year 2000: Use By Normal Humans*. W.D. Evans and N.S. Kline, eds. Springfield, Ill.: Charles C. Thomas, 1971, pp. 109-127.
13. Rothman, D. Behavior modification in total institutions. *Hastings Center Studies*, 5:17-24, 1975.
14. Wilkins, L. Putting treatment on trial. *Hastings Center Studies*, 5:35-48, 1975.
15. Lehmann, H.E. Speculations on use of psychotropic drugs in gerontological practice. In: *Psychotropic Drugs in the Year 2000: Use By Normal Humans*. W.D. Evans and N.S. Kline, eds. Springfield, Ill.: Charles C. Thomas, 1971, pp. 53-68.
16. Gottschalk, L.A. The use of drugs in information seeking interviews. In: *Drugs and Behavior*. L. Uhr and J. Miller, eds. New York: Wiley and Sons, 1960, pp. 515-519.

17. Gottschalk, L.A. The use of drugs in interrogation. In: *Manipulation of Human Behavior.* A.D. Biderman and H. Zimmer, eds. New York: Wiley and Sons, 1961.

18. Sedgwick, P. Illness—mental and otherwise. *Hastings Center Report,* 1(3):27, 1973.

19. Laing, R.D. *The Politics of Experience.* New York: Ballentine, 1968.

20. Siegler, M., and Osmond, H. *Models of Madness, Models of Medicine.* New York: Macmillan, 1974.

21. Szasz, T. *Ideology and Insanity: Essays on the Psychiatric Dehumanization of Man.* Garden City, N.Y.: Anchor Books, 1970.

22. Barber, B. *Drugs and Society.* New York: Russell Sage Foundation, 1967.

23. Freedman, D.X. Drugs and culture. *Triangle,* 10:109-112, 1971.

24. Freedman, D.X. The social and psychiatric aspects of psychotropic drug use. In: *To Live and To Die: When, Why and How.* R. Williams, ed. New York: Springer Verlag, 1973, pp. 227-239.

25. Klerman, G. Psychotropic drugs as therapeutic agents. *Hastings Center Studies,* 2(1):81-94, 1974.

26. Klerman, G. Psychotropic hedonism vs. pharmacological Calvinism. *Hastings Center Report,* 2(4):1-3, 1972.

27. Lennard, H., et al. *Mystification and Drug Misuse.* New York: Harper & Row, 1972.

28. Veatch, R. Drugs and competing drug ethics. *Hastings Center Report,* 2(1):68-81, 1974.

29. Donaldson, K. *Insanity Inside Out.* New York: Crown, 1976.

30. Foucault, M. *Madness and Civilization.* New York: Vintage Books, 1973.

31. Goffman, E. *Asylums.* Garden City, N.Y.: Anchor Books, 1961.

32. Rosenhahn, D. On being sane in insane places. *Science,* 197:250-258, 1973.

33. T. Scheff, ed. *Mental Illness and Social Processes.* New York: Harper and Row, 1967.

34. F.J. Ayd, ed. *Rational Psychopharmacotherapy and the Right to Treatment.* Baltimore: Ayd Medical Communications, 1974.

35. Shader, R., and DiMascio, A. *Psychotropic Drug Side Effects.* Baltimore: Williams and Wilkins, 1970.

36. Swazey, J. Chlorpromazine in psychiatry. In: *A Study in Therapeutic Innovation.* Cambridge, Mass.: MIT Press, 1974.

37. Gallant, D. Essay on boundaries between research and therapy. Prepared for the National Commission for the Protection of Human Subjects of Biomedical and Behavioral Research, 1976.

38. Jonsen, A. Do no harm. In: *Philosophical-Medical Ethics: Its Nature and Significance.* S. Spicker and H.T. Engelhardt, eds. *Philosophy and Medicine,* Vol. III, D. Reidel. Holland: Dordrecht, 1977.

39. Ingelfinger, F.J. Informed (but uneducated) consent. *New Eng. J. Med.,* 287:466-470, 1972.

40. Laforet, E.G. The fiction of informed consent. *JAMA,* 235:1579-1585, 1976.

41. *Cobbs v. Grant,* 502 P. 2nd 1 (Cal. 1972).

42. Katz, J., and Capron, A.M. *Catastrophic Diseases: Who Decides What?* New York: Russell Sage Foundation, 1975.

43. Jonsen, A. A map of informed consent. *Clin. Res.,* 23(5):277-279, 1975.

44. Downie, R.S., and Telfer, E. *Respect for Persons.* New York: Schocken Books, 1970.

45. Harris, E. Respect for persons. In: *Ethics and Society.* R. T. de George, ed. Garden City, N.Y.: Doubleday, 1966.

46. Kant, E. *The Groundwork of the Metaphysics of Morals.* H.J. Paton, trans. New York: Harper Torchbooks, 1974, pp. 64-74.
47. MacLagen, W.G. Respect for persons as a moral principle. *Philosophy,* 35:193-217, 1960.
48. Williams, B. The idea of equality. In: *Philosophy, Politics and Society.* P. Laslett and D. Runciman, eds. Series 2. Oxford: Blackwells, 1967, p. 116.
49. Klein, D., and Davis, J. *Diagnosis and Drug Treatment of Psychiatric Disorders.* Baltimore: Williams and Wilkins, 1969, pp. 20, 23.
50. Holder, A. *Medical Malpractice Law.* New York: Wiley and Sons, 1975, Chap. 1.
51. Locke, J. *Second Treatise on Human Nature.* P. Laslette, ed. New York: Mentor Books, 1965, p. 311.
52. S. Hirsch, ed. *Madness Network News Reader.* San Francisco: San Francisco Glide Publications, 1974.
53. American Medical Association. *Principles of Medical Ethics,* No. 6.
54. Burrows, J. *AMA: Voice of American Medicine.* Baltimore: Johns Hopkins University Press, 1963, Chap. 9.
55. Willis, J. *Clinical Psychiatry.* Oxford: Blackwell, 1976, p. 2.
56. Redlich, F., and Mollica, R. Overview: Ethical issues in contemporary psychiatry. *Amer. J. Psychiat.,* 133(2):125-135, 1976.
57. Perelman, C. *The Idea of Justice and the Problem of Argument.* London: Routledge and Kegan Paul, 1963.
58. Rawls, J. *A Theory of Justice.* Cambridge, Mass.: Harvard University Press, 1971.
59. Rescher, N. *Distributive Justice.* Indianapolis: Bobbs-Merrill, 1966.
60. Vlastos, G. Justice and equality. In: *Social Justice.* R.B. Brandt, ed. Englewood Cliffs, N.J.: Prentice-Hall, 1962, pp. 31-72.
61. *In re Joseph Lifchutz,* 2 Cal. 3d 415.
62. Summary Report of Task Force on Confidentiality of the Council on Professions and Associations of the American Psychiatric Association, 1975.
63. *Tarasoff v. Regents of the University of California,* 33 CA3d 177.
64. Davis, A., et al. *Schizophrenics in the New Custodial Community.* Columbus: Ohio State University, 1974.
65. Strauss, A. *Chronic Illness and the Quality of Life.* St. Louis: C.V. Moseby, 1975.
66. Greenblatt, M., et al. *Drugs and Social Therapy in Chronic Schizophrenia.* Springfield, Ill.: Charles C. Thomas, 1969.
67. Ban, T.A. *Schizophrenia, A Psychopharmacological Approach.* Springfield, Ill.: Charles C. Thomas, 1972, Chap. 2.
68. Garber, R.S. The impact of psychopharmacology on medicine and psychiatry. *Psychosomatics,* 11(5):386-390, 1970.
69. Crane, G.E. Clinical pharmacology in its 20th year. *Science,* 181:124-128, 1973.
70. Kline, N. Manipulation of life patterns with drugs. In: *Psychotropic Drugs in the Year 2000: Use By Normal Humans.* W.D. Evans and N.S. Kline, eds. Springfield, Ill.: Charles C. Thomas, 1971.
71. Merloo, J. Medication into submission: The danger of therapeutic coercion. *J. Nerv. Ment. Dis.,* 122:353-360, 1955.
72. Szasz, T. Some observations on the use of tranquilizing drugs. *Arch. Neurol. Psychiat.,* 77:86-92, 1957.
73. McCormick, R.A. The moral right to privacy. *Hosp. Progress,* 57 (8):38 ff., 1976.
74. Fletcher, J. Ethical aspects of genetic controls. *New Eng. J. Med.,* 285:776-783, 1971.

75. Olin, G.B., and Olin, H.S. Informed consent in voluntary mental hospital admissions. *Amer. J. Psychiat.*, 132:938-941, 1975.
76. *Winters v. Miller*, 446 F. 2d 65 (1971).
77. Halleck, S.A. Legal and ethical aspects of behavior control. *Amer. J. Psychiat.* 131:381-385, 1974.
78. Gallant, D.M. Psychiatric treatment of the lower socioeconomic classes. *News of the LPA*, 5:1-3, 1966.
79. Jonsen, A.R., and Hellegers, A.E. Conceptual foundations for an ethics of medical care. In: *Ethics of Health Care*. L. Tancredi, ed. Washington, D.C.: National Academy of Sciences, 1974, pp. 3-21.
80. Barber, B. Liberalism stops at the laboratory door. Presented at the American Sociologic Association Meeting, San Francisco, Aug., 1975.

CHAPTER VI

Concluding Remarks and Recommendations

DONALD M. GALLANT AND ROBERT FORCE

At this time, we would like to thank all the contributors for their thoughtful and interesting remarks. The presentations were predictably of high caliber and the commentaries exceptionally stimulating. It appears to us that such discussions not only clarify problems but also generate new ones, many of which are solvable. We would like to make some specific recommendations which we hope will prove helpful to further the ethical conduct of both research and psychiatric practice.

ETHICAL CONDUCT OF RESEARCH

1. A central clearinghouse for Institutional Review Boards (IRBs) or Human Research Committees (a much more appropriate term) should be established for collection and dissemination of various IRB decisions that may set helpful precedents for other review boards. In addition, such a clearinghouse could help in the exchange of information between the individual IRBs. It is also proposed that a regional hierarchy of IRBs be established for those cases warranting appeal by either the clinical investigator or institution.

2. Governmental support for the training of patient surrogates should be initiated immediately on a trial basis after the establishment of standards and objectives to guide the individual patient surrogate. These patient surrogates should be used only as *advisors* to certain specific groups or individuals:

177

those especially vulnerable populations residing in poverty areas, prisons, and mental institutions, and families of those patients with limited mental capacities. The surrogates would serve as *decision-makers* only for those individuals with limited mental capacities who have no available families. The surrogate should be utilized on a protocol-by-protocol basis and not be regarded as automatically required for these classes of people. Otherwise, the existence of a surrogate would only detract from the dignity of the patient and create another impossible bureaucracy.

After a reasonable period of time has elapsed, the surrogate program should be evaluated to determine whether or not the goals have been achieved.

3. The independence and competence of IRBs or Human Research Committees should be increased as follows:

a. All competent researchers should be required to rotate as members of the committees.

b. Those members of the Human Research Committees who are laymen should be required to have practical didactic and experiential training in the medical-legal aspects of research and be financially compensated for their time.

c. A professional patient surrogate should serve as an advisor to each Human Research Committee.

d. The Human Research Committee should have indemnification from law suits.

e. Periodic evaluations of IRBs by inspection teams of peers and governmental personnel should be conducted. These evaluations should be made according to published, predetermined criteria.

4. The National Commission for the Protection of Human Subjects of Biomedical and Behavioral Research should apply federal regulations to *all* research conducted in the United States.

5. All medical schools that receive any type of federal financial support should be required to conduct adequate courses in the ethics of research.

6. Regulations in regard to Phase I studies, mental capacity requirement for consent without proxy, and consent problems in children should be clarified. For example, with children seven years of age or older, not only is proxy consent required, but these children themselves are required to sign consent. It is quite apparent that there are many children in this age group who do not have the ability to comprehend informed consent in research or treatment and their written agreement is farcical. The requirement that drugs used in Phase I studies in children must have first been proved to be safe in adults is a blanket requirement which is not always appropriate. For example, if it had been necessary to establish the safety of Ritalin in adults prior to use in children, a number of adults would have become habituated and addicted without the associated therapeutic benefit. An observation of adult addiction

to Ritalin has no relation to the use of Ritalin in hyperkinetic children where addiction potential is minimal to absent.

Regulatory agencies and courts need legal doctrines to guide them in resolving intrafamily disputes concerning appropriate proxy consent for research and treatment with individuals who have only a limited mental capacity to understand informed consent. One of the reasons for conflicting court opinions has been the use of the framework of therapeutic versus non-therapeutic research rather than the more basic question of "degree of risk."

7. Patient surrogates should always be available if any one of the three basic requirements of informed consent are not present: (a) the mental capacity and comprehensive ability to give consent; (b) voluntariness or free unhampered choice; (c) sufficient knowledge of the research protocol to give informed consent.

8. A gradual effort should be made to establish basic minimum requirements for researchers who perform their work on human patients.

9. For more competent and efficient testing of a drug during the early phases, the FDA should contract with hospitals associated with medical and research institutions for such studies. These institutions should be carefully evaluated and then selected for the conduct of Phase I and Phase II studies. Thus, the early research would be concentrated in research units which can be easily investigated and evaluated on a frequent basis and conducted by reliable, competent individuals.

10. Every scientific journal should require that the submitted manuscripts describing human experimentation should detail the manner in which informed consent was obtained. Thus, we disagree with Beecher's recommendations that the manuscript should not be accepted for publication if the details of the informed consent described in the paper are inadequate. If the details of informed consent are inadequate or deleted, the author should be requested to complete this section. If the informed-consent procedure is truly inadequate, the manuscript should be published with a criticism of the informed-consent procedure following the article in the same medical journal. In this manner, those studies that did not utilize adequate informed consent would not be allowed to go undiscovered because they were refused publication in a journal. In addition, the patients in this study would not have exposed themselves to risk in vain.

ETHICAL CONDUCT OF PSYCHIATRIC PRACTICE

1. A stricter regulation of institutional standards for licensure by federal as well as state agencies should be a requirement for all institutions to remain open for patient care. Inspection should be made by teams of peers as well as federal and state personnel to help guarantee adequate treatment. The ques-

tion exists as to whether or not the Joint Commission on Accreditation of Hospitals (JCAH) should be utilized for this licensure since it may be more subject to political pressure and may have more of a self-serving orientation than a federal agency.

2. Human Rights Committees should be established on a trial basis along similar guidelines as those described in the *Wyatt v. Stickney* decision, except that it would be our hope that these Committees would be somewhat more flexible in their orientation toward treatment settings. A working association between the physician, institution, and the Committee rather than an adversary relationship would eventually result in more efficacious and adequate treatment for the patient.

3. A central clearinghouse should then be established for all of the Human Rights Committees for collection and dissemination of Committee decisions that may help set helpful precedents for later treatment problems that may arise.

4. As outlined in the previous section, the use of patient surrogates should be made available to these treatment institutions and Human Rights Committees as they would be available to the IRBs.

5. The Human Rights Committee should have a number of members who should be required to have practical didactic and experiential training in the medical-legal aspects of treatment and be financially compensated for their time. In addition, all competent physicians should be required to rotate as members of these Committees. Such efforts would help to increase the competency of these Committees and enable them to function in a more adequate manner.

6. All medical schools should be required to conduct adequate courses in ethics of treatment.

We realize that there are many additional suggestions of help to the physician-scientist as well as to the patient-participant in both research and treatment. However, until the above minimal recommendations are achieved, genuine reform of our medical research and treatment system is unlikely, and advances in both competent research and treatment will be hindered.

Index